The

LONGEST
MILE

The LONGEST MILE

A DOCTOR, A FOOD FIGHT,
and the FOOTRACE THAT RALLIED
A COMMUNITY AGAINST CANCER

CHRISTINE MEYER, M.D.

SHE WRITES PRESS

Published 2016
Printed in the United States of America
ISBN: 978-1-63152-043-3
Library of Congress Control Number: 2015954802

Cover design by Julie Metz Ltd./metzdesign.com
Cover photo by Jamie Stanek
Interior design by Tabitha Lahr

For information, address:
She Writes Press
1563 Solano Ave #546
Berkeley, CA 94707

She Writes Press is a division of SparkPoint Studio, LLC.

Names and identifying characteristics have been changed to protect the privacy of certain individuals.

Never doubt that a small group of thoughtful, committed citizens can change the world. Indeed, it's the only thing that ever has.

—Margaret Mead

For my husband, Chris
Because he makes me better

In Memory of Ed Kokoszka 1959-2016

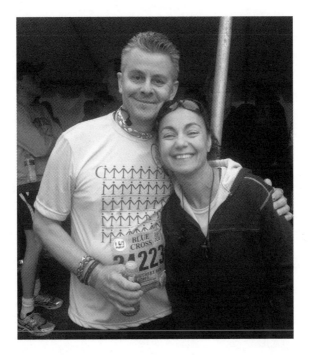

The 2016 Team CMMD Broad Street Runners dedicate their 3000 miles on May 1, 2016 to Ed Kokoszka. Ed was a beloved member and mentor since the inaugural Broad Street Run on May 5, 2013. He was an avid runner and had finished the Broad Street Run over twenty times. Although Ed lost his life suddenly on December 13, 2015, he will forever be a part of Team CMMD.

CONTENTS

Chapter 1: HADER YA HABIBTI

Love is composed of a single soul inhabiting two bodies.
—Aristotle

It was one of those brutally hot July days in Philadelphia. When I left my office at 5:00 P.M., the heels of my ridiculously impractical shoes virtually sank into the melting asphalt. As usual, my Wednesday as an internist had been long and stuffed with patients in every available moment. I had not had time to pee, much less eat lunch. A massive pile of papers on the desk had looked particularly intimidating as I shoved it into my briefcase. About a month later, I would find one of my kids' report cards in a patient chart—a casualty of the turmoil that was my life.

Nonetheless, Wednesdays were actually my favorite day of the week. Even though they were universally and mercilessly busy, I took solace, as I chugged through patient after patient and call after call, in the fact that my husband, Chris, was home. *It's all good*, I told myself over and over again. These three words were essentially the "deep breath" that calmed me, no matter what cacophony of ringing phones and chattering patients was unfolding around me. By the time I crawled through the door on any given Wednesday, my husband would have seen that the kids had practiced music, dinner was waiting, the counter had been scrubbed, and all three children had done an extra hour of algebra; even our youngest, five year-old Hadley, got variables drilled into her head on Wednesdays. Walking into my warm house to find moaning children being lorded over by their smug father almost always erased the trauma of my workday from my weary mind, and I would spend the evening basking in that comfort.

Chris was the anchor in our house. His easy smile and quiet steadfastness balanced my fast-paced, no-time-to-rest persona. My husband of sixteen years was the only one in my life capable of calming me no matter what I might be worrying myself into a frenzy about. If I tossed and turned at night about a sick patient, he would turn on the light, pull me close, and say, "You will do your best, like you always do. She's lucky you are her doctor." When I called him from my car, breathless and panicked at my uselessness as a mother, after our daughter Maisy's first public temper tantrum, he laughed a little first, then said, "Just be firm and calm and stand your ground. You are a great mom; she's just a normal three year-old!" When the eye doctor told us that our son, Sam, then just four, needed glasses, I wept—he had gotten my vision. Chris put Sammy on his back and piggybacked him around, looking for the coolest Spider-Man frames. He had a way of making any news seem not so bad. With him, I could handle just about anything.

That particular Wednesday, as my face met the inferno of

the outdoors, I saw Chris's tall, lean shape emerging, almost on cue, from the haze of the summer sun. His gait was always relaxed and casual. Years of running and hiking had given his strong legs a saunter that seemed effortless. But not that day. Although he was coming toward me quickly, there was nothing light about his step. On the contrary, I thought I detected the slightest hitch in his long stride, as if he were a bit reluctant to close the space between us.

My smile faded as he neared. His perpetually happy face was drawn. When he was just an arm's length away, he reached for me. He was steadying me for something about to hit hard.

"Cat," he said, "your aunt is sick. She just had emergency surgery. I don't know a lot, but it sounds pretty bad."

The words tumbled down like rocks on the slide. I had four aunts, but Chris did not have to tell me which one had brought him to me that day. The sick, empty feeling in my stomach, the sudden loss of power in my legs, and the agonizing heaviness in my heart identified her for me. From my father's youngest sister, whom I called Tant, I learned about kindness, compassion, and deep, unconditional love of family. Tant loved people in general, but she especially loved her "boys." Her husband and two sons were everything to her. My swimming thoughts instantly went to Uncle Stephan, Jack, and James. I thought of their big, ground-shaking steps and bigger, soul-warming laughs. I pictured their dining room table and saw Uncle at the head. Tant was always to his left, and Jack, their oldest son, at his right. James sat next to his brother. And my spot was to Tant's left. I spent a decade at their dinner table. No matter what happened, those positions never changed.

With searing clarity and undeniable guilt, I found myself

thinking about the food on that table, too. Tant, as busy and gifted a physician as she was, cooked dinner for her family practically every night. At such a moment, hearing she was so sick, I should not have been thinking about food. And yet it was all I could do to push the recipes and images and smells out of my head. After a moment, I stopped trying and let my thoughts of Tant's cooking challenge my disbelief and grief. Her food back then, and my recollections of it at this moment, brought me comfort—no dish more so than her *rozz*.

This plain rice can take side stage as a bed for slowly stewed vegetables in a rich tomato gravy or shine in the national dish *koshari*, a savory pilaf of rice, lentils, fried onions, and macaroni. When guests are expected, nothing is considered more fitting for an occasion than *mahshi*, whole vegetables, such as peppers, eggplant, and zucchini, hollowed and stuffed with a mixture of ground meat, onions, and, of course, rice. No matter what the final result, virtually every Egyptian dish starts with or includes basic *rozz*.

I first learned this recipe when I was about ten years old. We were in Tant's first apartment in New Jersey. She had not been in America long and still cooked very much like her mother did: with a passion and tenderness that people could practically taste—even in her simple pot of rice. Tant pulled up a small stool for me to stand on and handed me one ingredient at a time, coaching me step by step. She let me melt the butter, stir in the noodles and rice, and pour the water. She taught me to taste the cooking liquid and adjust the salt. In the end, she bragged, "Catty made the *rozz* all by herself!"

It was one of my proudest moments—not only did I make an entire pot of rice, but she called me Catty. I loved when she called me that. Christine was long and so very "English." Catty, Cat, Cat-coota—those names she had for me rolled right off her tongue and wrapped around me like a warm blanket.

That night at her dinner table, my aunt smiled broadly as my uncle exaggerated the deliciousness of what had always been Tant's specialty. "Your aunt has some competition in the kitchen now!" He laughed.

She made *rozz* the same way every time and always in the same imported stainless steel pot. That French vessel itself reminded me of her: gleaming, graceful, and ever so slightly rounded on the bottom.

Uncle Stephan loved to tell people that he married Tant for her voluptuous figure and her irresistible cooking. He was so much like a father to me that when I called him Uncle, it was with the same tone I would have used for my dad.

Until I practically lived with them, I did not understand the concept of a husband and wife cherishing each other. She was just nineteen when they met, and a good eleven years Uncle's junior. Despite being an intimidating man—big, tall, smart, successful—he looked at her as if she were the only thing that mattered to him in the entire world.

Hader ya habibti was my uncle's most often uttered phrase. Literally translated, it means, "Yes, my love."

Whether she was asking for a glass of water, a swimming pool, or a condominium at the beach, his response was the same: *hader ya habibti*. Sometimes he said it tongue in cheek, sometimes in all sincerity, but always with a twinkling smile that belonged to her and only her.

Every morning for decades, she brought him coffee, and every morning, without fail, he thanked her with that look—as if she had just given him an unexpected treasure. Even when they disagreed, their tone was never disrespectful or angry. In the end? *Hader ya habibti.*

* * *

Now, as Chris delivered the bad news, I crumpled to the curb, sobbing. When I was finally able to compose myself, I made some barely coherent phone calls. Detail by detail, the pieces of Tant's story came together with agonizing certainty.

She had been sick for a while—at least six months. If I had been speaking to her regularly, I would have known that. But I hadn't called in a long time. It wasn't that I didn't care to or want to; it was just that life had gotten in the way. I would get busy with charts or e-mails or paperwork and just forget.

Despite the fact that I adored her and that she was the single most influential person in my life, I felt as if I had abandoned her. My stomach turned. Suddenly, I was five again, in my grandmother's posh apartment in Cairo. It was the summer of 1977 and stiflingly hot. As was customary in Egyptian immigrant families, I had been sent to Egypt with a family friend to live with my grandmother and aunts and uncles for two years. My parents were working night and day, trying to realize the "American dream" that always seemed just out of their reach. My father had rented a storefront in a terrible part of town. He stood for twelve or fourteen hours a day, waiting for a customer. It would take decades for Americans to understand and seek out Middle Eastern groceries and delicacies. Back then, his aching back and worn shoes resulted more from waiting *for* customers than from waiting *on* them.

My parents' knowledge that I was safe with my father's extended family allowed them to toil on, just until they had enough money to move out of their roach infested walk-up in Jersey City, New Jersey, the city where nearly all Egyptian immigrants settled. My father always wanted a house with a huge yard where he could try to grow Egyptian vegetables, which he planned to sell to Americans. The least expensive land and homes were found in sleepy towns deep in the Pine Barrens of South Jersey. Being able to buy a house on a couple of acres of land would mean that my parents had finally achieved success.

Ironically, before my father immigrated to the United States, his family was already enjoying the wealthy lifestyle he was now scrambling to achieve. The three-story building they owned housed four apartments: three rented ones and a huge three-bedroom, which they occupied. The solid brick construction and wall-to-wall marble floors kept the interior of the building surprisingly cool, despite the absence of air conditioning. Hand-forged wrought-iron gates wound their way around the circular staircase and along the plentiful balconies, which overlooked the bustling sidewalk markets below. Fresh fruits and vegetables were piled high on wheeled wagons. An old man, Assad, dressed in a djellaba, a long cotton dress, peddled freshly picked and washed bundles of arugula and juicy watermelon.

To avoid repeated treks up and down the marble staircase, my uncles rigged a large, hand-woven basket to one of the balconies. They would take my grandmother's carefully penned lists and lower them to the man on the sidewalk. Assad would load the groceries into the basket and give the rope a quick tug, indicating to my uncles that the basket was ready. They always threw in a few extra cents for his trouble.

On this day in 1977, we had just eaten crusty French bread, still warm from the bakery, and mortadella, along with fresh tomatoes that had been hoisted up in our handy basket. After lunch, the grown-ups retreated to the sitting room for tea and biscuits. I hated that sitting room with the fancy chaise lounge and miserably uncomfortable chairs. A virtually identical Queen Anne settee was mandatory in every Egyptian immigrant household in Jersey City—only in Cairo, they didn't bother with the permanent plastic covering. It was just too hot for plastic.

In my bare feet, I tiptoed down the cool, dark marble hall to my favorite place in the huge apartment: my aunt's room. Tant was sitting on the floor. The milky skin of her face was scrubbed clean. She smelled like soap. A long cotton skirt was tucked around her crossed legs. She was surrounded by preserved human bones. Papers and open textbooks littered the hand-knotted Persian rug.

She was so engrossed in her work that at first she did not notice me. I stood for a second and then started to fidget—a little too obviously—hoping she would look up. Tant promptly obliged. She gave me a giant, warm grin and patted the floor in invitation. As I plopped down happily next to her, she handed me a large, long bone. I ran my finger over its many ridges and grooves, just as she did. Years later, I would learn that it was a human femur—the largest bone in the human body. Tant was in her early twenties, and at that time, I didn't understand that she was studying to be a doctor. Yet it was at that moment, watching her caress the huge thigh bone, that I knew: someday I would do exactly what she was doing.

The more curious I became, the more time I wanted to spend with Tant. She lived her life in the same systematic way in which she had studied those bones: routine after routine. It was in those routines that I was created.

Her mornings always started with the strongest Turkish coffee—serious coffee. The fine grounds always settled to the bottom of the glass. A spoon standing straight up in those grounds was the sign of a proper cup. My aunt and uncle sipped from those small, pungent glasses as if they had all the time in the world, while they chatted about the day ahead and chuckled quietly at the craziness in store for them.

Tant was a natural beauty. Her smoky blue eyes seemed to change color with her mood. Crystal clear meant she was happy and relaxed. Cloudy and dark meant she was worried. I especially loved her hair. Her thick braid reached the middle of her back. It reminded me of a warm, setting sun—not blond, not brown, but somewhere in between. She had to split it into sections to brush it. Before she discovered that Americans paid for curls like hers, she spent hours beating them out. As she got older, her hair got shorter. And yet, no matter how short it was or what color or style it was, it always seemed to suit her angular face.

She was meticulous in her appearance. Her clothes were always in the latest style and yet professional and conservative. No one would ever have known by looking at her army of shoes—which were never sensible and *never* flat—that she spent fourteen hours on her feet every day.

As an internist, she was responsible for caring for patients in the hospital, as well as in her office. When I was old enough, I was allowed to go along with her on hospital rounds. I always seemed to have to run a little to catch up to her *click-clacking* heels. She walked with purpose. It was instantly obvious to anyone who saw her coming that she knew exactly where she was going and what she was going to do when she got there. It was the same walk in the hospital, in her office, or in the meat aisle of the local grocery.

As Tant made her way to the first patient room, an invisible crowd parted for her. Nurses, respiratory therapists, and unit clerks all moved ever so subtly out of her way, all the while smiling warmly. They all loved her. The minute she crossed over the threshold into her patient's room, time stood still. She had arrived where she was needed. No matter how busy she was or how late she was running, she would take her coat off, put her purse on the chair, and settle herself comfortably on the edge of the bed. Tant would then open the stuffed three-ring binder that held patient medical charts long before electronic medical records and quietly study report after report. No one in the room spoke until she looked up. It was always her patient whom she looked at first. It did not matter that some of them couldn't meet her gaze. Whether she was delivering good news, bad news, or no news at all, she managed to bring comfort to patients and families with just that one look.

Tant always touched her patients, even when she wasn't examining them. She would hold their hand, squeeze their shoulder, or rub their back. I must have subconsciously learned to become a "toucher" from her. *My* touching was more of a nervous tic than an instinctive act of comforting, though; I tended to give a gentle slap on the back after listening to a patient's lungs or a quick pat on the knee after checking a reflex. My look-touch-examine-slap pattern turned disastrous once after a complete—and I mean *complete*—physical on a male patient. Once I had thoroughly inspected his rectum and declared his prostate healthy, I delivered a no-holds-barred, full-on, palm-down, red-mark-leaving slap on the gentleman's bare ass. It was not my proudest moment. Telling Tant that story made her giggle, even as her cheeks turned pink.

With her own patients, she closed her eyes as her stethoscope made contact with their chest. There were only three things in the world at that moment: her, the patient, and that most critical, rhythmic sound. When she stood up, she would straighten her clothes and smile down. No matter the outcome of that visit, everyone involved was just happy she had been there. I felt lucky just to be near her.

* * *

Chris was squeezing my shoulder now, standing over me as I cried and rocked on that scalding curb. As he reached down for me, his sad eyes told me to go. He checked the gas gauge and reminded me to fill up. Then he kicked my tires and hugged me to him.

"Be careful. I love you, Cat," he whispered.

The trip from my office to the hospital in New Brunswick would take me at least an hour and a half. I turned the radio off and on and off again. I cried and laughed and shook my head as memories of my *tant* and our years together filled my mind. I remembered how tiny her waist looked in her starched white coat. I remembered how she leaned the small of her back against the wall as she listened intently to the patient in front of her. I thought of her slow blink and deep inhalation that always signaled a moment of concentration. I remembered her laugh, her eyes, and the way she twisted her wedding band on her thin finger over and over again when she was nervous.

Then, just like that, an hour and a half had passed and I was there. Having spent the last fifteen years of my life in and out of hospitals, I did not expect to feel scared when I arrived at St. Peter's that night. As it turned out, I was terrified. The old volunteer at the information desk handed me a visitor's pass and said, "She must be some great lady; she has had so many visitors!" I hated her for saying that. My aunt's having many visitors was a terrible thing—it meant she was sick enough to be here. She was sick enough to *have* visitors.

The elevator door opened onto a bustling medical world I had spent days and nights and years in, and yet I felt completely out of place. I hated the noises. I hated all the beeps and buzzes and indecipherable overhead pages. The smell of antiseptic mingling with that of human excrement turned my stomach. At every nursing station I passed, the cast was the same: weary nurses slurping old coffee from flimsy Styrofoam cups.

The incessant ringing of phones complemented the droning. Whatever that person on the other end of the line was calling for could not have been as important as my *tant*. How could people be sitting, eating, chatting, and calling, when she lay there so sick? *How dare they interrupt my grief-stricken walk down this endless hallway?* I thought.

She was in the last bed in the corner of the intensive care unit, but when courage finally willed my shaking hands to pull back the curtain, I did not see her at first. On the buzzing radiator, a half-eaten doughnut lay against a still-full cup of Dunkin' Donuts coffee. It had been there a while. That cold cup of American coffee was nothing at all like the coffee Tant and Uncle drank. It did not belong there in that room. I wanted to reach for it and fling it down the hallway and as far away from Tant as I could.

The woman lying on the bed was thin, frail, and pale. She looked so small—like the bed itself might swallow her up. There were tubes erupting from her arms, her nose, and her bladder. My once beautifully accessorized Tant was now adorned with nothing but a thin hospital gown. Her feet—usually crammed into the most fashionable of shoes—were now held hostage by compression boots. Their periodic inflation managed to startle me even after the tenth time. In place of her necklaces and bracelets lay oxygen cannulas and IV tubing. I squirmed a little at the sight of the Foley catheter draining urine from her bladder. *She hates that thing*, I thought with authority. At the sight of clear yellow urine filling the bag, I let out an audible sigh. *Her kidneys are good.* And yet everything was wrong.

The private room did not provide much respite from the beeps and buzzes of the ICU hall. They came from the heart monitor and blood pressure cuff and IV lines. She could barely turn her head, but she knew I was there. Her eyes grew wide. I was already weeping. I leaned in to kiss her cheek and hug her, but I ended up lying on top of her. So many things strapped her down that I could not get my arms around her. "I am so sorry," I cried over and over again.

I was sorry that she was sick and in pain. I was sorry that I hadn't called. I was sorry that it had taken this to get me to her. I was sorry that I hadn't been there for her. Maybe if I had, she would have told me she hadn't been well. Maybe if I had called, I would have heard the ever-so-slight weariness in her voice. I would have asked her questions—good questions—just like she had taught me to. I would have found out that she never did get that colonoscopy. I would have convinced her to. I would have been the kind of doctor she inspired me to be—the kind of doctor *she* was.

When I finally pulled myself off of her, she smiled feebly at me. "I'm fine," she whispered. "Don't worry. I'm fine."

But I knew she wasn't fine. I knew because even as the words left her mouth, a single tear rolled down her cheek. Somehow I knew she wasn't crying for herself; she was crying for us—her family, her sons, and especially her husband.

It was not until that day in the small, dark ICU room that I really understood the meaning of the word "anguish." There sat Uncle, squeezed between the window and the commode she was too sick to use. He looked smaller than I remembered. His eyes, which always seemed to beam sharply and thoughtfully, suddenly looked lost. And when the weight of it finally was too much, he did something I had never seen him do: he put his drawn, contorted face in his hands and wept. As the sobs racked his body, a single lock of his carefully combed-over hair fell across his brow. And there it stayed. Because for the first time ever, my *tant* did not have it in her to reach over and push it back into place.

Chapter 2: BACK IN THE GAME

Whether you think you can, or that you can't, you are usually right.

—Henry Ford

The notation on my schedule said simply, *Patient just wanted to see you.* I felt my stomach tighten and my hands go numb, and before I could stop myself, I thought, *Cancer.* In the months after Tant's diagnosis, the disease, in all its different forms, seemed to have taken my practice hostage. I no longer enjoyed patient visits and in fact seemed to drag myself through most days with a vague sense of dread—uncertain of what blow the next patient would deliver to my already-fragile psyche. Some days seemed to bring a whole parade of cancer sufferers through my doors. On this bright September afternoon, Joe Dunn came to see me for the last time.

Joe was sitting on the exam room table, shrunken and pale. Despite his emaciated face and atrophied legs, his belly pulled his black T-shirt so tight that it seemed to be trying to escape. At his feet lay a black duffel bag. I crossed the space to where he sat and threw my arms around him. I did not need him to recount for me his recent treatment failures; I knew all about them. It had been a brutal eight-year fight. When he was my age, forty-two, Joe had been diagnosed with Stage IV colon cancer and given less than six months to live.

Despite his dismal prognosis, he had a lot to live for: five kids, to be exact. Joe's twins were just three when he was diagnosed. He kept those little girls in his sights and absolutely refused to give up. He had years upon years of unending chemo. He had surgeries to remove lesions from his liver and endured months in and out of hospitals.

But, as Joe often reminded me, those eight years of treatment hell were punctuated by graduations, award ceremonies, concerts, and wrestling matches. He had taught his younger son to drive and had just seen his other son off to college when the wheels started coming off his treatment plan. While lying in bed one night, Joe turned on his side and heard a pop. With that tiny movement, his clavicle had snapped. After he spent several weeks in the hospital, it became apparent that the treatments were finally failing and Joe was going to die.

As I pulled away from him, he began to cry. He looked at me pleadingly. "I don't want to die, Christine."

I handed him a Kleenex. Eleven years of higher education and nearly thirteen years of clinical practice, and all I could offer my dying patient was a tissue.

He saw me awkwardly stepping over the duffel bag and answered the question I had been afraid to ask. "It's a change of clothes," Joe explained. Over the last few months, his sick, swollen, failing sphincter had become less and less reliable. He never knew when he might have an accident, so he had gotten in the habit of carrying clean clothes everywhere he went. As if the inescapability of his numbered days, the pain of snapped bones, and the torment on his wife's face were not enough, Joe also had to worry about soiling himself in public. "Today is going to be a long day," he said softly—the implication being that he might need more than one set of clean clothes.

He explained that his wife and kids had been through enough. He could not leave *anything* for them to take care of. Over the years, he had steadfastly kept up his life insurance. His personal finances were meticulously organized. He had shown his oldest son how to use their tractor mower. Five handwritten letters addressed to each of his children lay on his desk. There was one last appointment on his calendar. From my office, Joe was heading across town: he had funeral arrangements to make.

A few weeks later, I learned that Joe had opted to go on hospice. His in-home nurses specialized in end-of-life care and would see to it that he was comfortable in his last days. I signed orders for morphine to ease the pain, alprazolam for anxiety, and low-flow oxygen for respiratory distress.

I leaned heavily on the granite countertop as I gave my receptionist Joe's papers. "Fax these for me?" The few sheets seemed to weigh fifty pounds, as it required palpable effort for me to hand them over. Samantha gave me an apologetic glance and then presented me with an updated copy of my daily schedule. My normally upright, fast-moving frame was all but curled up in front of my star receptionist.

"I put her in at the end of the day—so you would have time . . ." Samantha's voice trailed off awkwardly, acknowledging that no explanation was necessary. Debi McLaughlin's name on the schedule printout caused my heart to sink. How was it possible that cancer had managed to get this sweet, loving mother and wife in its grip, too? Debi was less than a year older than I was, yet I was allowed to live and she was not.

I remembered the day, ten years before, when we had met. She had come to see me when she was heavily pregnant with twins and had ended up delivering them later that day, after I sent her to labor and delivery straight from my office on account of her very high blood pressure. From the day those babies were born, we were forever "office" friends.

Although we never saw each other socially, she visited me regularly, never missing a physical or a required checkup. Over the years, her family grew. Invariably, she had a kid or two with her at our visits. I never minded. In fact, I sometimes took comfort in kneeling down to chat with one of them. It made the fact that I was hours from seeing my own babies easier to take.

Despite the passage of time and both of our increasingly busy lives, Debi and I remained close. Ever since the life-or-death moment that had thrown us together, Debi and I had had a bond far stronger than that of a typical doctor and her patient. Plus, she was easy. Debi never got sick. Often, nearly a year passed without our seeing each other. But whenever we reconnected, it was as if time had stopped. Her easy smile and her adoration of her five kids made Debi my hero. Seeing her name on my schedule used to put an instant hop in my step. Not so this day, though. I sucked in a deep breath that seemed to burn its way deep down into the pit of my stomach.

It had been less than a year since Debi was diagnosed with cancer. In early 2012, she dutifully came in right on time for her annual exam. She was one of the patients I always greeted with a hug, and that day was no different. She smiled at me warmly, and we immediately launched into the continuation of a conversation we had started months before. As I moved systematically through her exam, we talked about our five-year-old girlie girls and how both of our boys seemed to need remedial shoe tying.

I will never know whether my friendship with Debi cost her her life.

Months later, I would repeatedly run through that last exam. If I hadn't been chatting, would I have noticed something? Was there the slightest drop in her weight? Did she have the littlest shadow under her eyes? Was that freckle different? On Mother's Day 2012, just months after her annual physical, without warning, Debi lost vision in her right eye. After a series of emergency appointments at WillsEye Hospital, she was diagnosed with choroidal carcinoma, a rare but aggressive melanoma that had originated in a tiny freckle in her eye.

Debi dove freely and fearlessly into her treatment plan, enduring painful laser treatments to her eye. She spent her days going between scans and doctor's appointments. During the day, I stood by as faxes with her name on them rolled onto my desk. Melanoma notoriously spread to the liver and brain, so the finding on Debi's liver MRI that "multiple small lesions were present and could represent metastasis" sent waves of terror through me.

The radiologist was right in his assessment that "metastasis could not be ruled out." In fact, those tiny spots quickly became large and innumerable. Chemotherapeutic drugs were directly injected into Debi's liver circulation, in the hope that they would target the cancer cells without damaging her liver. These treatments were repeated countless times. Each time she was admitted for chemo-embolization, she tolerated the aftereffects of nausea, diarrhea, and vomiting less. Debi often remained dehydrated and weak for days afterward. In the end, the grueling treatments were successful at only one thing: systematically destroying Debi's liver.

I saw her in my office right after one such treatment. She came in hanging onto her husband. She was thin and weak. Her skin was a sickening and unnatural yellow, as if she had accidentally fallen into a vat of PAAS Easter-egg dye and hadn't pulled herself out quite in time. Her right eye was no longer able to focus. She was dehydrated and sick and desperate to avoid yet another trip to the hospital. If I could just give her a bag of fluids, maybe I could reverse the spiral of dehydration, nausea, and further dehydration. I stuck her seven times in an attempt to place an IV that day. She lay quietly and let me. I knew I could do it. I knew I could get that IV in. Maybe then she would walk out of my office stronger. Maybe she would be less yellow. Maybe she could tuck her kids in that night. Maybe her cancer would go away. The utter fantasy of my IV-placing skills was only slightly less ridiculous than my last hope.

Of course, none of those things would happen. Finally, I gave up on the IV catheters and gave Debi a small antinausea pill to put under her tongue. When it finally kicked in, she was able to drink a small bit of water. As I walked her out to my waiting room, I made her promise to call me overnight if she felt worse.

My futile attempts at putting in her IV had caused me to be

over an hour behind in my schedule. As irritated patients eyed me over the tops of hopelessly outdated magazines, I heard Debi call softly, "Christine?" I ignored the angry stares and walked over to her. She put her hand on my cheek and stared at me with her one good eye. I didn't realize it till later, but Debi must have thought that would be the last time I saw her alive.

She was saying goodbye.

While Debi was gathering the devastating facts of her disease and then bracing for the road ahead of her, my aunt was being told she needed a minimum of six months of chemo for Stage IIIB colon cancer. The morning of that day in July when I found out she was sick, she had woken up in severe abdominal pain. She was never one to complain, so when she insisted that Uncle drive her to the emergency room, he did so without hesitation. Much later, Tant learned that the tumor had perforated her bowel. Although the normal human colon is full of good, protective bacteria, a perforation and leakage of those bacteria almost always cause a life-threatening infection known as peritonitis. Without immediate surgery and antibiotics, Tant faced certain death.

When she had recovered her strength, she told me of her late-morning trip to the emergency room. The ER doctor thought it would be fine to send her home with a diagnosis of stomach flu.

She argued with him. "No. I have peritonitis. I know it. You have to admit me. Call Dr. Jacobsen, the general surgeon. Tell him I'm here."

Because she was one of the few internists who still rounded on her patients in the hospital, all of the ER doctors knew and respected her. Soon after the ER physician called him, Dr. Jacobsen arrived. He was scrubbed and Tant was prepped for the operating room within hours. Sadly, the peritonitis was good news relative to the large colon tumor that had caused the perforation in the first place. As only she could, Tant turned out to have saved her own life.

Over the next few weeks, every night I sat in my car, summoning the courage to dial my aunt's home phone number. Uncle would pick up, and I would sit silently as he called, "Hello? Hello?" The minute the words "How is she?" left my mouth, I sobbed uncontrollably. Nothing I said from that point forward was coherent or useful, but he let me say it—time after time, evening after evening, week after week. Occasionally, he would summon Tant. Her weak laugh would start me sobbing all over again. "Stop!" she would insist. "I'm fine. I'm fine."

* * *

One bright Tuesday morning, about a month after Tant's surgery, Chris woke me up with a gentle kiss and a pat on my shoulder. "Honey," he said, shaking his head a little, "did you hear the massive storms last night?"

I nodded sleepily, fighting the urge to yell at him for waking me up to tell me about the torrential downpours we had just had.

"Um, well, you didn't put the BMW in the garage . . . and you left the sunroof and windows open. There's about six inches of water on the floor of the car. I threw some towels in there, but you're going to need to try to dry it out."

I sat up on my elbows and watched him walk out of the bedroom, still shaking his head. I buried my face in my pillow to stifle a giggle. His pants were sopping wet from the hem to a third of the way up his calf, and yet, as he always did, Chris just brushed off the ruined car, wet pants, and derailed morning and walked out with a smile.

Technically, leaving the windows open during a downpour did not qualify as a "distracted driving" problem—I was just distracted, period. However, a few days later, when we learned that my little act of "forgetfulness" had resulted in the insurance company's declaring a "total loss" of the very expensive vehicle, Chris just tacked it on to all of our other automotive mishaps and concluded that, really, I should not be allowed to own, much less drive, a car. After the BMW incident, I promised him that if I ever found myself getting into, getting out of, or driving a motor vehicle, I would focus solely on that vehicle: not my phone, the radio, or anything else.

The hardest thing of all for me to control, however, was my brain. The most egregious distractions were my own unstoppable, racing thoughts of Tant, patients, tumors, treatments, and, most of all, my growing list of failures.

The afternoon after my attempts to give Debi IV fluids was no different. My mind was turning with the events of the day. I thought of the poison she was enduring and the damage it was doing to her body. I thought of her littlest daughter, who would never remember her mom should she die now. I thought of my utter uselessness as a doctor to my friend.

As I wiped stinging tears from my eyes, I spotted a runner out of the corner of my eye. The sight of the young man's bright orange shorts, and his T-shirt peeled off his glistening chest and rammed into his pocket, caused my heart to jump. His appearance on the shoulder of that busy road reminded me of two things. First, I had, once again, been distracted and had not seen him until I was practically right next to him. And second, I really needed to start running again.

* * *

By the time Debi and Tant were diagnosed, I had been running for five years—since just after Hadley, my youngest, was born. While my third pregnancy was relatively uneventful, the days after her birth were the most stressful of my adult life—that is, until Tant got sick. Hadley arrived in an operating room much like her older brother and sister: on time, by scheduled C-section, head perfectly shaped, having been spared the travel through the tortuous birth canal. As my incision was being closed, I craned my neck to peek at my new baby in Chris's arms. I was looking for the dazed, dreamlike smile he always seemed to have whenever he was caught holding a baby, which, given his job as a pediatrician, was practically every day. But he wasn't smiling. In fact, that day, his face had the same drawn look it did when he came to my office to tell me Tant was sick.

"What's wrong? What's wrong with my baby?" My voice sounded as heavy and useless as my epidural-paralyzed legs, but my brain was screaming for me to run to him, to snatch her out of his arms, to fix whatever was causing him to make that face.

No one answered me for what felt like hours. Finally, they brought her over. There was another doctor now, one I didn't know. But she knew Chris. He let her speak.

"We have to take little Hadley to the neonatal intensive care unit [NICU] for a bit," she said. "She's having some trouble breathing, but she's fine. We just need to get her some oxygen."

Chris's face told me they did not just need to give her some oxygen. As I sobbed, he leaned down and put his face so close to mine that our foreheads touched.

"Listen to me, Cat. Our baby is going to be fine. She is breathing fast probably because she came a few weeks too early. Her lungs weren't quite ready."

He wiped my tears with his hand, a hand that always took bad away and left good.

"You promise?" I asked.

"I promise," he said without blinking or hesitating.

I knew Chris meant what he said, but things didn't work out that way. The night after Hadley was born, I was awakened from my narcotic-induced sleep by a gentle tap on my arm. In the dark, I could make out only a small figure in scrubs. Chris was on a cot next to me. He went from lying to standing in a second when he saw that it was Dr. Murphy, the neonatologist from the NICU.

It was 2:00 A.M. Terror passed through me like an electrical current, searing and numbing at the same time. Hadley had a collapsed lung. The doctors needed to perform an emergency needle decompression to remove trapped air from outside her lung in order to allow it to fully expand again.

Chris and I scrambled down to the NICU; I was oblivious to the pain in my belly, and Chris was oblivious to everything around us. Dr. Irfan was going to assist Dr. Murphy in the procedure. He had done his residency with Chris and greeted him like an old friend.

As he slapped Chris on the back, he called out, "Man, you gotta see this X-ray—it's a total whiteout!"

Dr. Irfan made this announcement with the same exuberance he might have used to call out a football score.

Shut your stupid mouth! I screamed in my head. I couldn't believe how cavalier Dr. Irfan was being about something so catastrophic. There was nothing cool about a whiteout X-ray—all it said to me was that my baby's lung had collapsed completely.

Chris shot me a knowing look, signaling that I needed to keep it in, and shook his head quietly.

"No, thanks. Can you just let us know when the procedure is over?"

Fortunately, the needle decompression was successful and Hadley's condition improved rapidly, but the next nine days were still agonizing. Despite the fact that she was a big, healthy-looking baby, Hadley's lungs were not mature. They called it respiratory distress of the newborn—a condition that carried an excellent prognosis. Statistically, with time, Hadley would in fact be just fine. But all the terminology and statistics did not matter to me then. I sat next her tiny crib, staring at indecipherable monitor screens and flinching at every beep.

In those seemingly unending hours of waiting, I thought back on my pregnancy with unbearable guilt. This distressed newborn was my baby girl, and I had caused her distress because I had not had the sense to stop working. Whenever my pregnancy seemed to get in the way of my work, I made an accommodation—anything to avoid taking time off. When waves of nausea gripped me unpredictably, I designated one exam room for "puking only." That way, if I had to suddenly excuse myself from a patient room, I would not have to walk far to get to a sink. When sciatica numbed my right leg to my toes, I brought in a stool so I could hoist my ailing, massive thigh onto it in an awkward half-sitting, half-standing position. When my feet swelled over my notoriously high shoes, I switched to flats. When my lab coat wouldn't button, I left it open. Even though it was obvious to everyone around me that I was getting bigger, slower, and more tired by the minute, it never occurred to me to stop working. Not being there for my patients was not an option—no matter what.

*   *   *

Finally, the longest nine days of our lives were over. Chris's tall frame crouched over the tiny car seat, fussing with the five-point harness. After checking and double-checking, he was satisfied that our baby was secure and we made the much-anticipated trip home. It had been ages since I had prayed, but that morning I stared out the car window, ignoring the jabs of pain every road bump sent through my healing belly, and repeated over and over, "Thank you, God. Thank you, God. Thank you, God."

Once we were settled, I spent entire days sitting on the couch with Hadley in my arms. I stared at her nose and did not have to wonder whose it was—it was button-shaped and slightly upturned, exactly like Tant's. I stroked her cheek over and over, mesmerized by its flawlessness. I never wanted to put her down. Hadley's birth and NICU ordeal seemed to have lengthened my notoriously short temper. In fact, with her in my arms, I could not imagine being angry at anything again.

So I shocked myself when, during one such motherly moment, Chris came bounding down the stairs, dressed in running shorts and shoes, and I found myself wanting to throttle him. It started innocently enough: he bent to kiss Hadley on the forehead and gave me a warm look, ignoring my Coke-bottle glasses. He patted my unwashed hair and made no comment about the fact that I was still in my nursing nightgown at 4:00 in the afternoon.

"Hey! I'm going out for quick five-miler, okay?"

It was absolutely not okay. I felt fat, bloated, and exhausted. The trauma of Hadley's first few days of life, coupled with my surging and crashing hormones, had left me emotionally spent. I did not want him to go for a run. I did not want him to be dressed and chipper and awake and lean. I wanted him to sit on the couch next to me and be fat and bloated and mentally drained, too.

Chris must have read my mind, but instead of unlacing his shoes and putting his arms around me, he said the unforgiveable: "Hey! Come for a run with me! We can put the baby in the jogging stroller. My parents won't be back with the other kids for hours."

Only my years of utter adoration for him kept me from blurting out the profanities raging in my head. I made no effort to move and just stared at him blankly, as if I could not even bother to acknowledge the stupidity of his suggestion.

He persisted: "Trust me. You will feel so good afterward."

I wept as I yanked open drawers, searching for some semblance of exercise gear that would fit over my still-gigantic belly. Finally, I settled on an old pair of Chris's scrub pants. I grabbed a pair of scissors and, with little decorum, cut them off at the knees. His Ben & Jerry's Cherry Garcia T-shirt barely stretched over my girth, but it would have to do. My old sneakers felt two sizes too small, so I gave up on the laces and stomped down the steps, counting the minutes until my little exercise in marital support would be over. I was angry at Chris for implying that I needed to move, that exercise would be good for me. And I was especially angry because I could not shake the feeling that there was some truth in what he was saying to me.

Chris pushed the baby jogger, walking first, then gradually picking up speed, all the while looking back at my scowling face with a smile. It was late July 2007, and the air felt as deep and wet as a lake.

"Come on!" he called. "Just run a few steps, then walk a few. Run a few, walk a few."

I did it only because I believed him. I believed him just as I had that day Hadley was born when he'd told me she would be fine. Deep down, I knew he was right.

I made it only a third of a mile that first day, but when we got home, I felt about a hundred pounds lighter.

Over the coming weeks, Chris and I went out for "runs" together several times. With every outing, I ran a little farther and felt a little better. One day, I noticed that I was actually able to lace up my shoes, as the fluid in my feet had finally gone down. Once I could no longer cinch the scrub pants tight enough, I switched to old yoga pants, and when they started to slip off, I rewarded myself with my first pair of actual running capris. I ran in our neighborhood and I ran on the treadmill. I even started running alone.

While it would take me months to admit it, Chris had opened up a new world for me—one that would ultimately save me and change the lives of forty-seven strangers.

Chapter 3: FAILING

When you die, it does not mean that you lose to cancer.

You beat cancer by how you live, why you live,

and in the manner in which you live.

—Stuart Scott

I quickly learned that I am not alone. In fact, most amateur runners have a compulsive mental disorder. Fortunately, it manifests itself only in the last hours before a race. Suddenly, *that* run is the most important thing in the world. You feel like if you miss it or if you are late or if everything doesn't go according to plan, the world just might end.

I believe this has to do with the tremendous emotional and physical energy runners invest in their race training. By the time race day actually happens, most runners have spent weeks or months running regularly, according to a tight training schedule. In those weeks, we have great runs and then, seemingly without reason, we have terrible runs. We applaud ourselves for getting out there and getting it done; then—sometimes even on the same day—we berate ourselves for being slow and tired. We make excuses for not running and swear we are hanging up our shoes, when suddenly we have breakthroughs—moments of cool breezes and warm sunshine. In those moments, we feel as if we could run forever.

And then, just like that, the training roller coaster is over and the night before the race is upon us.

* * *

After I started running with Chris, one fact emerged as indisputable: not only did running consistently help me lose baby weight and improve my sleep and energy levels, but it also had a dramatic impact on my state of mind. In fact, Chris's dragging me out on that first run after Hadley was born most certainly cured a case of postpartum depression I had been somewhat in denial of. When the daily stressors of managing my house, job, practice, and kids weighed me down, even a short jog around the neighborhood lifted my spirits.

I had been running consistently for two years when I registered for my first official race. Chris was running a half marathon in Philadelphia over Thanksgiving weekend of 2009. Along with this popular 13.1-mile race, there was a shorter, five-mile run. After a few of our runs together, Chris printed out a training program called Couch to 5K. It promised to turn any couch potato into a runner capable of completing a 5K run (3.1 miles). The eight-week plan required a commitment of just three thirty-minute sessions per week for two months. I pinned the sheet to the wall next to our treadmill and taped a Sharpie marker underneath. Every time I finished a session, I crossed it off the page with gusto. Before I knew it, the sheet was covered in giant black Xs and I was a 5K runner.

On my own, I managed to push myself to run 3.5 miles, but in my brain a wall went up right there. I was not made to run more than 3.5 miles—no way, no how. But after I saw the notification about the five-mile option during Chris's race, it occurred to me that if I registered to run five miles, I would be forced to actually *prepare* to run five miles. Using the techniques I learned from Hal Higdon and his Couch to 5K program, I built my own schedule with more boxes waiting to be Xd out.

I was not confident enough to run outside for five miles, though. So, instead, I got on my treadmill and set the workout time for sixty minutes. My goal was to be able to finish five miles before the treadmill shut off at the one-hour mark. There were days when I felt like a Clydesdale, trudging along on stumpy legs. There were days when I slammed off the power button on the treadmill because I was disgusted with my lack of progress. I covered the display with a towel so I wouldn't look at it, only to throw the towel across the room . . . right before throwing it in. It was agonizing.

Then, just weeks before the race, it happened. I was watching *Top Chef* on the basement TV and was so engrossed in the show that I didn't realize I had been consistently increasing the speed on the treadmill—the set pace had seemed a little too . . . *easy?* The episode ended. Sweat dripped down my nose and onto the display. I wiped it away with my hand and blinked. I had done five miles in fifty-seven minutes. I felt shocked, elated, and proud. But most of all, I felt ready.

Chris's parents had volunteered to take the kids for the weekend, so we had decided to stay in a hotel the night before the race. Parking and traffic are a nightmare in Center City, Philadelphia, on any given day, but race weekends brought the humming city streets to a standstill. The fact that the race start line was just steps from the Four Seasons Hotel made it an ideal spot for our night in the city.

After check-in, Chris whistled his way around the well-appointed room, digging through his small overnight bag and trying to recall whether he had packed socks. "Huh—you think the concierge has any?" Then he looked at my bag and laughed. "Well, *you* certainly have enough socks there, don't you? You know it's only *one* race, right?"

I couldn't even look at him. I, on the other hand, had packed three different pairs of socks in all different thicknesses. I had scoured four weather sites for the race-morning forecast and tested out both long-sleeved and short-sleeved running shirts, before settling on the former. With an almost superstitious tenacity, I had insisted on packing the exact clothes—down to the underwear—that I had trained in. I was not about to try new shoes or socks or even a new bra on race day.

At dinner, I picked at my big plate of pasta, while Chris decided on a huge burger and two beers. I shook my head as he scarfed down the more-fat-than-carbs meal.

After dinner, we headed back up to our room. "Can you set an alarm for five?" I asked him.

"You realize it's going to take us four minutes to walk down to the start from here—and the race starts at eight, right?" Chris was smiling that smile, the one that let on that he knew I was being crazy but he loved me anyway.

I must have looked wounded, because he quickly followed with, "Well, actually, I did see a ton of runners staying here; the elevators might get tied up."

Chris sat up in bed, watching me from over the top of his book without saying a word, as I began systematically laying out my gear. Capri pants: check; well-worn running bra and old-lady panties: check (I wouldn't get up the nerve to run commando for a few more years); long-sleeved running shirt with moisture-wicking technology: check. I charged my phone, which would double as my music source, and slipped it into my armband. I tested the headphones to make sure both worked and fit snugly in my ears. Last, I pinned my race bib to the front of my shirt. I smoothed it with my hand. *I am actually going to do this. I am going to run in my first race.* My heart pounded and my stomach flipped. Despite the fact that this race was inconsequential, I was undeniably nervous. *Fifty-seven minutes. That's all you have to do,* I reminded myself.

To eat or not to eat right before a run had been a big source of anxiety for me. But, after several "dry runs," I had figured it out. I needed to drink one-half cup of coffee with a little cream and a tiny sprinkle of sugar. More, and I would have to pee; less, and I would get a headache. The best prerun breakfast for me turned out to be half a cup of corn flakes barely moistened with a splash of 1 percent milk. More, and I would get nauseous; less, and I would get hypoglycemic. It had taken me two years and countless runs to sort out those details.

I panicked as I looked through the in-room dining menu. No corn flakes. With shaking hands, I dialed room service.

"Well, of course, Dr. Meyer. We will be happy to send up

corn flakes. . . . Um, yes, of course, we will be sure to send up only half a cup. Yes, ma'am. One percent milk. Yes. It will be there by 6:30 A.M."

As I got underneath the plush comforter, I ran through my checklist one last time and finally drifted off into a fitful sleep. All night I dreamed of running naked or shoeless. I dreamed I came in dead last, just ahead of the street sweeper, and then I dreamed that I ran so fast I actually caught a little air.

When the alarm went off at five in the morning, Chris kicked me in the shin and groaned. I jumped out of bed the way I did as a resident when my beeper went off in the middle of the night.

I was dying for more than one-half of one cup of coffee. My head was caught in a vortex of sleepless exhaustion and excited anticipation. Upon checking into our room at the Four Seasons, we had found a basket of fresh fruit, granola bars, and water. The handwritten note from the hotel manager said, "Good luck in your race tomorrow! Please let us know if we may be of service!"

That morning, the fruit basket and the note lay next to the gleaming silver room service tray. The polished carafe of steaming coffee was surrounded by all of the items I had requested: corn flakes, milk, half-and-half, sugar, and ice water. I finished the half cup of coffee in two swallows and shoved the tray outside the hotel room door. I knew if it sat in the room, I would drink more coffee and my entire race-day plan would certainly unravel.

Sometime around 7:00, Chris and I walked down to the start line, holding hands and surrounded by hundreds of other runners who all seemed to be spilling out of hotels at the same time. Chris pulled me close to him. His strong arms, wrapped tightly around me, warmed me down to my toes in the chilly fall air.

"I am so proud of you." Chris's crystal-blue eyes gave me a look I knew well. It was the same look Uncle Stephan gave Tant. At that moment, even though Chris had his own, biggest run to finish, I was the most important thing to him. I knew it from that look.

"I don't want you to go. My stomach hurts!" I didn't even try to conceal my whiny tone.

"You are so ready for this, you have nothing to be nervous about . . . but for God's sake, stop farting—these poor people all around you!"

As he sauntered off, looking as if he were going to fetch a gallon of milk, not run thirteen miles, I could see Chris shaking his head and laughing. I could still feel his arms around me until he was out of sight. Then I stood there alone as my stomach churned, cringing at my uncontrollable gassiness.

It was a bright, sunny morning without a cloud in the sky, but it was cold. I hopped around from one side of the street to the other, chasing the sunny patches to keep warm. I watched as the elite runners—those expected to finish in record-breaking time—took their place just behind the start line. Those runners were not jumping around from one sunny spot to another. In fact, I had seen them sprinting up and down the road minutes before, "warming up." I could not imagine spending one ounce of my energy doing that before running the actual race. In fact, I believed that I really needed to conserve every single step and contemplated sitting down right there on the sidewalk so that my "standing" wouldn't use up all of my running mojo.

Michael Nutter, the mayor of Philadelphia, was the emcee.

"All right, runners!" he called from his perch on the raised platform just to the side of the start line. I was too far back to see him, but his words carried clearly over the humming crowd.

"This is a glorious morning for a run! A 'zero excuses' kind of day!"

Runners around me fiddled with their headphones and arm straps. Some were on the ground, stretching one last time. I just wanted to run. I didn't bother to check my headphones or my laces. The thought of stretching on the ground, in the middle of the massive crowd, terrified me. I would be the runner pictured on the front page of the newspaper the next day for having been tragically "trampled because she was too slow to get up when the gun went off."

The starting gunshot startled me and sent the elite athletes flying down the road. The throng of runners around me erupted in applause. Because of the massive number of participants, we were queued behind the start line for a few blocks. It would be several minutes before the regular runners even got *to* the line.

Finally, we began moving up the block. A brisk walk gave way to a trot and then a full-on run as we crossed over the start mat that would link to the computer chip embedded in our bibs. Even though the gunshot had started the race twenty minutes earlier, official times were recorded from the moment a runner's bib crossed over the start line. I slammed my right foot down onto the thick rubber mat. *You have totally got this. Fifty-seven minutes. That is all,* I told myself over and over.

After a few minutes, my mind and stomach began to settle down. My dollar-store headphones had gotten hopelessly tangled in my back pocket, so I tossed them to the side of the road. For a moment I felt guilty about my flagrant littering but quickly shoved the thought aside. I would not be able to hear my iPhone running app tell me how fast I was going, but I quickly shoved that panicked thought to the side, along with the headphones, and I suddenly felt liberated.

Once I stopped worrying about my absent headphones, my loose shoelace, and my slipping sock, I found my groove. My breathing slowed down, became regular, and seemed to keep time with the runners' feet all around me. I suddenly remembered advice that Chris had given me a few weeks before. "Don't forget to look up!" he had said. Until then, I had been staring down at my feet and the road right in front of me, but the minute I heard his voice reminding me to look up, the running suddenly felt effortless. I felt as though an invisible rope connecting my belly button to the finish line was towing me. I stopped feeling the pain in my right knee and ignored the blister on my left foot where my sock had slipped down. I moved along, amazing myself with my rhythmic, confident gait and steady breathing. My arms pumped up and down, helping to propel me along city block after city block.

In my mind, I started to write the life story of every runner I passed or who passed me. *She's young, probably a runner in high school. Bet her parents are at the finish line. That guy . . . he's hurting. Wonder if he's ever run five miles before. Wow. Look at her! I'm going to try to keep up with her; she's about my age and has big thighs, too! Forget that. She is going very, very fast.*

Suddenly, I found myself practically on top of a gigantic blue sail marked with 2 MILES. I couldn't believe it. I had barely done the mental math, trying to calculate my pace, when I found myself next to the three-mile marker. I gave up on the pace calculation and just accepted the fact that the race was going so fast, I was well over halfway done and had never felt better.

Meanwhile, the crowd had become thick and boisterous. I high-fived a little girl sitting in her stroller and imagined she was my own little two-year-old, Hadley. Tears stung my eyes. But, to my surprise, they were not tears of pain or exhaustion or fear; they were tears of pride.

Before I knew it, the finish line was in front of me. And rather than crawl over it, as I had imagined I would, I sprinted with all my might—racing toward the end like a mother to her lost child. When I came to a stop behind hundreds of other finishers, my legs were shaking. I had to lean forward to catch my breath. My head swam with feelings of relief and joy. All around me, runners were collecting their medals and clear plastic bags stuffed with coupons for running shoes, water bottles, and granola bars. I felt as accomplished as if I had won the entire race. I wanted to dance and cry and jump up and down but felt silly doing so alone.

Chris would not be done for a while. As I walked back to the hotel to wait for him, it occurred to me that I had no idea what my finish time was. I felt certain of one thing: my pace must not have been very fast, because by the end I had felt as good as I had after my easiest, slowest runs.

I was already naked and just about to step into the shower when I remembered that I could get my finish time instantly by scanning the code on my race bib with my iPhone.

It took just seconds for it to pop up: 48:13.

There had to be a mistake.

I had finished five miles in forty-eight minutes and thirteen seconds? That meant each mile had taken me roughly 9.6 minutes. In all of my months of running and training, I had *never* run that fast, nor had I ever felt so good at the end of a run. *That* was the definition of "race-day pace"—and I had discovered it accidentally! It was then that I understood for the first time that if I wanted to keep running, I had to keep *racing*. And to keep racing, I had to keep training. I *needed* the motivation of a scheduled, committed race to motivate me to train diligently.

After that first race, I ran consistently, peppering my year with 5Ks and even the Broad Street Run, a ten-miler, in 2010. Little did I know, when I finished that race in an hour and thirty minutes, that it would plant the seed of another, life-changing Broad Street Run attempt a few years later. After Broad Street, I told myself that a half marathon was really just a ten-miler plus a quick 5K tacked on at the end, and in late 2011 I finished the Philly Rock 'n' Roll Half Marathon in two hours and twelve minutes.

A few months after the Rock 'n' Roll Half, my longtime patient Rosella Washington came to see me for a "routine" visit. The first time I heard Rosella sing, the hair on the back of my neck stood up and tears sprang unwillingly to my eyes. She was a "belter." Despite the most delicate string instruments that accompanied her predominantly jazz band, Rosella was a powerhouse. Her voice was like a huge net. It seemed to carry for miles, roping in anybody in its path. Sad, scared, lonely, tired—any and all within the vast earshot that was her listening distance would be comforted by the mere sounds of her notes. The first time I heard her voice on a CD, I closed my eyes and imagined how she might look. Years later, when I met her for the first time, I stopped dead in my tracks. Her voice had painted her portrait to a T. She was a beautiful, larger-than-life woman. Her long braids were never out of place. She had eyes the color of tea that had steeped just a little long and that beautifully complemented her flawless, deep-brown skin.

Whenever I think of Rosella, I remember a simple gold cross she always wore. I knew her for nearly eleven years, and never once was she in my office without it. My aunt had taught me to close my eyes as I listened to a patient's heart. For scores of visits over the years, as I laid my stethoscope on Rosella's chest, that cross would lie right where my stethoscope needed to be. Just before my eyes shut, I would scoot it over just a hair and stare at it for a split second. On the bottom, there was a small loop studded with a few simple diamonds.

I would learn a lot about Rosella from that cross. First, she was very clean—not as in pure, but as in soap-and-water clean. Not only was that cross always on, but it always had the tiniest bit of soap stuck in its loop. You would have to be very close to Rosella to see it. I wondered who besides her husband and me got close enough to her to see that soap.

Second, Rosella was also one of the most faithful people I had ever met. She never took that cross off. Not for a shower or a doctor's visit. Not for anything. She spent her days devoting her gift to praising God. Every Sunday, she was the voice of her church worship. Several times a year, she sang to audiences packed with those faithful to her and to Christ. Even the skeptics couldn't help but close their eyes for a second and sway to her rhythm. If God existed in a singing voice, it was in hers. No matter what life handed her, she accepted it gracefully as God's will.

Then she got cancer.

That afternoon, we had finished discussing Rosella's mild diabetes and high cholesterol. Before her visit, I had been distracted by the news that my aunt had been readmitted to the hospital with severe abdominal pain and a high fever, but I did exactly as Tant had taught me: the minute my foot crossed into my patient's room, no one else was there or mattered. Having accomplished my objective to discuss diet and exercise for Rosella's mildly high blood sugar, I smiled gently at her in encouragement. "You can do this!" I said like a silly cheerleader. Just as my hand touched the door handle, she stopped me. I didn't turn to face her. The words she spoke had the exact same effect on me as the first words I heard her sing: the hair on my neck prickled. "Oh, hey, Christine, there's one other thing. . . . Mark would kill me if I forgot to ask you about this. . . . I found this lump under my arm. It doesn't hurt, really; it's just hard to sleep on that side."

Before I even laid a hand on her, I knew Rosella had cancer. Within weeks, it was confirmed that the lump under her arm was a cancerous lymph node. The primary site was Rosella's breast. The day she heard the news, she looked down at her lap and shook her head in disbelief. She had not missed a mammogram. In fact, she had even had an MRI. No breast cancer had ever been detected—until it turned up in that lymph node. Not only did she have metastatic breast cancer, she had the most vicious kind. Like Debi, Joe, and Tant, Rosella was now in the fight for her life.

Rosella spent exactly one year getting chemo and radiation. The breast lump was removed after the adjuvant therapy had caused it to shrink but, like Debi, she was really never free of her cancer. It marched along without mercy. The last time I spoke to her, she could barely talk, her lungs were so filled with cancerous fluid. The voice that once boomed with such strength as to shake walls, chandeliers, and disbelievers suddenly couldn't even whisper a full sentence. As quickly as it was drained, that poisonous fluid reaccumulated, and with every drop, her lung capacity shrank and her voice grew softer. That day on the phone, quiet as they were, the words she uttered were unmistakable. "I am not ready, Christine." She said it in the tone of someone confessing a sin.

Despite the strength of her faith, in the face of death, Rosella was afraid. No matter how dismal her prognosis or unbearable her pain, she never gave up. Instead, she kept looking for another angle, a different treatment, anything that would buy her more time. In that last conversation, she asked me to research clinical trials. I knew she was too sick to qualify for a study and yet I spent hours online and on the phone. I gathered data and organized a spreadsheet of details. Even as the futility of my actions pounded in my brain, I knew that I was giving Rosella the only thing I could: hope. False and unrealistic as it was, I sent it. I fired link after link and spreadsheet after spreadsheet to her with the same useless tenacity with which I had poked Debi's brittle veins.

In the months after Tant's diagnosis, Debi's cancer took over her liver, Rosella was literally drowning in the fluid that filled her lungs with the ferocity of an angry river, Joe was counting his days on Earth as he grew more and more weak, Tant was steadfastly accepting the poison administered through her veins every other week, and I began to find it hard to so much as breathe. Running became impossible. My running-gear drawer, previously in a perpetual state of half-openness, as I was always either taking things out or putting newly laundered items away, remained untouched.

One morning, I opened the drawer, pulled out a pair of running shorts, and had one leg in and one out when I collapsed against the dresser, sobbing. How could I possibly run? Running to nowhere seemed like the silliest, most futile activity I could engage in. The nerve I had even to consider a recreational run while Tant, Rosella, Debi, and Joe were in a race against time—a race for their lives. That morning, I kicked the drawer shut, angry at myself, both wanting to run and feeling absolutely incapable of running. My aunt, those patients, and the cancer chains that bound them to one another, to me, and to their inescapable fates invaded my every waking moment.

In fitful sleeps, I no longer dreamed of finish lines and flying. Instead, I dreamed of hair lost, eyes enucleated, bones snapped, and whispered pleas for mercy. My head throbbed, my stomach clenched, and my heart broke. I could hardly move some days. I forced myself out of bed and to work with a dread that began to overtake all of my waking moments. I stopped caring about the details and seemed, at least to many of my patients, to have become inattentive. In those months, I got more patient complaints then I had in all my years as a doctor.

One day I opened a letter from a patient, feeling in my gut that it was not going to be a thank-you note.

Dear Dr. Meyer:

Kindly release all of my medical records to Dr. Lavin Marks at Hillview Internal Medicine. I have decided to switch to a doctor who will actually care about my well-being. It was disappointing to me that Judy was more concerned with my CT scan findings than you, my doctor of seven years, were. I sincerely hope our paths never again cross.

Victoria Raines

My patients' opinions meant everything to me. And in Victoria's case, my opinion meant—or used to mean—everything to her. Years before, her rheumatologist had advised her to start medication for a severe case of rheumatoid arthritis. Despite the promise of relief from crippling pain in her hands and feet, Victoria refused to start that medication without talking to me first: "I will *not* take any medicine unless Dr. Meyer—*my* Dr. Meyer—says it's okay," she told the other doctor.

There was a time when Victoria Raines and thousands of other patients put their health and wellness in my hands with almost-blind faith.

That letter solidified it. There was no mistake. I, in all my forms—doctor, mother, wife, niece—was doing something I had never done before: I was failing.

As someone who had never failed so much as a spelling quiz, I found wrapping my brain around failing in medicine next to impossible. Throughout my training at Thomas Jefferson University Hospital in Philadelphia, an acclaimed teaching hospital, I'd learned that failing was what the *patients* did. They "failed" this treatment or that. They "failed" to respond to verbal and painful stimuli. They "failed" to thrive. Then there was the old, withering lady who had lain in the hospital for weeks on end without a single visitor. She was just "failing"—as in failing at life, winding down, calling it quits.

Now, for the first time in my career, failures were mine, not my patients', to own.

* * *

By then, it had been so long since I had run that I w__
sure I still could. The man I'd seen in the orange shorts on the
side of the road on my way home that day had been running as
hard and fast as he could. His face was contorted as if he were
in pain. He seemed to be running from someone or something.
He reminded me that I, too, needed to move and sweat and be in
pain—physical pain, not just the mental anguish that cancer had
inflicted upon me.

Around Thanksgiving 2012, for the first time in months, I
put on my running shorts and laced up my shoes. I didn't bother
with music or headphones. I don't even remember if I wore socks.
I just walked out the front door and started running. After the
first mile, I collapsed on a bench, barely able to catch my breath.
I gritted my teeth and cursed. *How could I let myself get so out
of shape?* I thought of Tant and her colostomy and the rice she
wasn't cooking and got up. I ran and ran and ran. I ran down the
hill from our house and did lap after lap in the neighborhood
park. I ran back up the hill and cursed every step. Then I did it
again and again and again. I tried to run the failures out of me.

I did not give myself a pep talk. Instead, I beat myself up silently. *You are ridiculous. You used to run a nine-and-a-half-minute
mile. Stop whining. You think Tant whines like this when she's on her
knees, throwing up after chemo? Do you think Rosella whines like this
when they're drilling holes in her chest to drain the cancer fluid? Do
you think Joe whines like this when one of his little girls climbs onto
his lap and says, "Daddy, I don't want you to die"? No. No, they don't.*

Maybe if I ran long enough, those failures would just ooze
out of my pores and evaporate with my sweat. Maybe if I ran
hard enough, something in my body would hurt me as much

as my aunt's colostomy hurt her or Joe's shattered clavicle hurt him. Maybe if my body hurt, it would take my mind off my breaking heart.

It was a long, punishing five miles that took me well over an hour to finish, but speed was the last thing I cared about that day. My knees and ankles were throbbing. My left shin was scraped from the base of my knee to the top of my foot after I stumbled coming up the hill. When I finally got home, sweat was drying in white streaks down my forehead and bloody scabs were forming on my shin. What I really needed was to sit in a tub of ice, but I settled for half a dozen Ziploc bags that I filled with crushed ice. I strapped one to each of my aching joints using ACE bandages, gauze, and, when those ran out, Scotch tape. I hobbled to the front porch, looking ridiculous, covered in random ice packs, face striped with dried sweat, soaking-wet T-shirt stuck to my back. As I collapsed into a white wooden rocker, I had a moment of blinding clarity. I *needed* to run like that. I needed something to train for. I needed a race.

* * *

About six weeks later, a couple of days after Christmas, we drove to Tant's house to pay her a visit. Tant had just spent a few days in the hospital, being treated for a wound infection. She was worn out from her surgeries and antibiotics and chemotherapy. She always sounded tired on the phone, and I couldn't remember the last time I had heard her laugh. I wanted so much to do something for her.

"I will cook for you!" I announced. "*Nefsik fi eh?* What are you craving?"

Tant was gracious but told me softly that she didn't even have a taste for her coffee anymore. She really couldn't think about food. That was a bad sign. That woman lived for her morning coffee with Uncle. If she wasn't drinking it, things were not going well. Tant emphasized that she really didn't want anyone to make a fuss. At that point, she was still getting chemotherapy. A port had been placed in her chest so that she would not have to keep getting new IVs. Every other week, on a Thursday, she would be connected to the lifesaving poison. It would burn through her thinning veins for hours. Afterward, while saline flowed through the same veins, feverishly rinsing them of the toxins, she would sleep.

Walking into her beautiful house that Saturday after Christmas, I was struck by several things. First, her home's cavernous interior would typically have echoed every sound: pots clanging, kids running, and phone ringing. That day, the house was silent. Normally, on a Saturday, Tant would be found prattling around in her kitchen, cooking for one of the several guests she was expecting that weekend. In the years before cell phones, she had perfected the ear-to-the-shoulder method of holding the phone while keeping both hands free to stir and chop. Since her phone rang multiple times an hour with patient calls, my uncle had found a cord that was over twenty feet long. Tant was almost always at the stove, phone to her shoulder, cord stretched. She did her two favorite things effortlessly and at the same time.

"No, no. You are not bothering me at all, *ya habibti*," she would coo into the phone to her patient. She called everyone *ya habibti*—my love. While she consoled, soothed, or advised, she cooked. Every now and again, Tant would motion frantically to my uncle to get something out of the oven or off a burner. She would wave and mouth silently to him, so as not to interrupt the patient rant she was listening to. He responded the same way to anything that she asked of him: he leaped up from whatever it was he was doing, happily at her beck and call.

Tant never seemed bothered by intruding phone calls even on her weekends. In fact, she seemed to enjoy them. And Uncle never seemed bothered by her interrupting him. He would accomplish whatever menial task she assigned him, lean over, and kiss her head gently. Then he would go back to whatever important work she had pulled him away from.

On that Saturday afternoon, the mandatory pot of rice was not perched in its usual spot on the stove. Tant was not cooking *rozz* or anything else, for that matter. Instead, she was sitting. After years of imploring her to "just sit down," I felt my heart break at the sight of her in that position.

She had not lost her hair, but she no longer had the energy to color and style it. That day, her curly gray locks were hastily pulled back into a short ponytail. The dark circles beneath her eyes revealed her exhaustion. A loose-fitting tunic and pajama pants replaced her usual smartly tailored outfit. There was only one reason she would be in such an outfit: she was trying to cover her colostomy bag. Against my will, my eyes wandered to the barely noticeable bump to the left of her belly button.

"I'm used to it now," she reassured me.

On this Saturday, December 29, 2012, as we chatted over tea and biscuits, Tant told us that she had only a handful of chemo treatments left. If the postchemo CT scans coming up were clear, surgery would be scheduled to reverse the colostomy that peeked out from her tunic. No one discussed what would happen if the scans weren't clear.

Two days after our visit, on New Year's Eve, I woke up feeling awful. I was frustrated, worried, and exhausted. It would be days before Tant would learn the results of her scans. I doubted I would even get dressed that morning, much less go to one of the several New Year's Eve parties to which we had been invited. Chris did not argue. He was just as content to stay home on such a cold, gray day.

As I absently stirred cream into my coffee, he wrapped his arms around my waist. The kids were still asleep, and the house was quiet. Chris pulled me to him and tightened the belt of my fleece robe, quietly endorsing my decision not to get dressed at all. He watched me trudge into the home office and wiggle the mouse of our family computer.

"Whatcha doin'?" he called. "Blogging?"

Just before Tant got sick, I had started a blog as a way to journal stories about the kids and our crazy work–home life balance. I called the blog *Despite My Medical Degree* and quickly learned that journaling not only helped me immortalize stories I cherished but also helped my patients relate to me. In the early months, the readership grew steadily, but the blog's true impact on my practice did not happen until that late fall of 2012.

Energized by my first run in months and inspired by my neighbors' enthusiastically stringing holiday lights on Black Friday, I had written a post about the fact that I really didn't like Christmas—that the holidays reminded me of darker times. Within hours, hundreds of people came forward in support.

"I hate Christmas, too!"

"I wish I could just wipe December off the calendar!"

"Thank you so much. . . . I was feeling like the real-life Scrooge! Glad to hear I am not alone."

That day, and again and again, writing my blog brought me comfort. The same was true of Facebook. I found that when I, a well-respected doctor in my community, shared an experience or a feeling that was unpleasant, an army of supporters always seemed to rally.

Thanks almost exclusively to Facebook sharing, my blog readership exploded and began averaging five hundred to one thousand views per day. New patients reported having chosen my practice because they found it refreshing that I was honest and "real."

"Wow! Doctors are human, too!" one new patient exclaimed. Facebook became a conduit between my patients and me, and eventually to a growing body of readers who weren't my patients. I put "it" out there and they embraced it, laughed about it, or cried about it, but ultimately the blog kept a conversation alive— a conversation that I personally and enormously needed.

Soon, I began starting and ending my day with a quick scroll through my Facebook news feed and blog statistics. I perused comments that had been submitted and conversations my posts had started. Some were inspiring, some scary, and others just left me shaking my head. Good or bad or in between, one thing became clear about Facebook: it was a guaranteed way to get a lot of information out to a lot of people in a very short time.

So that New Year's Eve Day, I wrapped my cold hands around my steaming cup of coffee and, like any self-respecting depressed person, logged on to Facebook to read about how wonderful everybody else's life was. I skimmed through post after post about New Year's Eve parties and bizarre, unrealistic resolutions. I scrolled through pictures of smiling families but felt weighed down by some invisible dark force. My head was stuck in a dark cloud of grief and frustration, as thick and gray as the midmorning winter sky. Every day people were dying from cancer. Every day new cancer diagnoses were being made. Cancer patients were getting younger, and their prognoses were growing more dismal. My aunt and my patients were suffering, and all I could do was sit back and watch. I felt trapped. My mind screamed for me to do something, but inertia paralyzed my body. Getting off Facebook, off the computer, and out of my robe would not fix a single cancer heartbreak.

I was deep into a *what does it matter, anyway?* thought when I remembered that brutal hill run from weeks before and was reminded that I needed to keep running like I had that day, despite the pain, because I needed to feel as if I was good at something. I knew that I couldn't save Debi or Joe or keep my aunt's tumor from growing back, and intellectually I knew I would never be able to run from the cancer that seemed to be all around me, but I needed to outrun the sense of helplessness that seemed to be overtaking me.

I don't know if it was an ad that I saw online or a link in a post. All I know is that the nine words practically leaped out of the monitor.

"Guaranteed Spots for Philadelphia's Broad Street Run—Register Now."

The Philadelphia Broad Street Run was an iconic race, famous for its flat, inner-city course—one that essentially takes runners on a historical journey through the heart of Philadelphia. Over the years, it had become known as the country's largest ten-miler. I remembered my first Broad Street Run, a few years before, and I just knew that the 2013 race would hold the cure for my own sluggishness, moroseness, and helplessness. What I wouldn't know until much later was that the 2013 Broad Street Run would not just save me but ultimately rally scores of cancer-weary people out of their own helpless fog.

Chapter 4: PERFECT EYEBROWS

Alone we can do so little; together we can do so much.

—Helen Keller

The year 2013 marked the Broad Street Run's thirty-fourth anniversary. The course was legendary for the thousands of spectators that spilled out from every neighborhood along the route, so much so that veteran and fledgling runners alike clamored for entry into the race. Over forty thousand participants were expected for the 2013 event. As a result, the race organizers had been forced to institute a lottery method of registration, which meant that wanting to—or, in my case, sorely needing to—run Broad Street did not guarantee a spot. According to the race website, registration for the lottery would not officially open until late February—a full seven weeks away. But as I kept reading, I discovered there was one way to guarantee a spot in the race at that very moment.

Charity teams running Broad Street to benefit select 501(c)(3) charities were exempt from the lottery. All members of these charity teams would be guaranteed a race bib. I gasped at the first charity I saw on the list, and the scalding coffee I was sipping found its way into my trachea.

The American Cancer Society: despite my choking, gagging coughs, it was in those four words that I found my answer. I would train for and run the Philly Broad Street Run in honor of Tant, Debi, Rosella, and Joe. As I browsed the site, I noticed that many of the registrants had formed individual teams for the American Cancer Society's running group, known as Team DetermiNation. Most of the teams were small—made up of five to ten runners. The rules were simple: Each member of a team had to raise $500 for the charity. In return, those runners would be guaranteed a bib for this sought-after race. Further, team totals were cumulative. If one person on a team raised $1,000, two runners on that team would earn spots. I had no doubt that I could do this run, but for the first time ever since I had started running, I did not want to run alone. I wanted a team. I *needed* a team.

As the possibilities circled in my mind, I felt my neck and face flush. The pale-blue, well-worn fleece robe I had vowed to spend the day in felt entirely too warm. I loosened the belt and shrugged it off. I needed room to pace, so I stood up, threw open the doors, and stepped into the foyer.

Chris was coming down the stairs. He looked past me, at the discarded robe lying behind me on the floor, and paused. "You okay?" he asked.

"I'm going to run Broad Street again!" I made the triumphant announcement as if I had just discovered the cure for cancer.

"Okay." He seemed shaken. In our twenty-some years together, he had learned that in my world, even the simplest task would take on life-changing momentum and that he would invariably, albeit unwillingly, be dragged along. "When did you decide to do that?"

"Two seconds ago." I gathered my heavy hair off the nape of my neck and piled it on top of my head in an expert bun held in place by the hair tie I always had on my wrist. I practically jumped up and down as I went on. "I'm starting a team—a charity team. We are going to raise money for the American Cancer Society."

Chris's smile started in his eyes and spread to his lips. His playful swat at my backside said it all. He knew running Broad Street for the American Cancer Society would be therapeutic for me. As we stood there in the foyer, both of us knew that for me to do this, what little free time I had would be devoted to training and fund-raising. While I lived with an avid runner, he could not be the first recruit on my team; I would need him at home.

I also needed a name for my team—something short, memorable, and catchy. I played with my aunt's initials. I browsed the Team DetermiNation site and was astonished at the wittiness of some of the team names there. Unlike the Buns on the Run or Too Inspired to Be Tired teams, everything I came up with seemed forced and unnatural. So I decided to set aside that task for the time being and focus on the actual bodies on my team.

After racking my brain for a few minutes, I sat down and tried to make a list but was able to come up with only three people whom I could persuade to join me: Tom Kuhn and Clare-E Nanacassee, two of my medical assistants, and Joan McFadden, the family doctor I had just hired to join my practice.

How could they turn down their boss—especially for such a great cause? In order for all of us to run the race, we would need to raise a minimum of $2,000. While that was certainly a respectable amount of money, it was also reasonable enough that if I had to, I could cover it myself. It seemed like a noble thing to do; plus, the guaranteed race entries, the motivation to do those long, cold runs in the winter, and the endorphins I so yearned for would be worth every cent.

The first thing I needed to do was to register my team in order to generate a link to pass on to potential teammates via my Facebook page and blog. I enthusiastically clicked the link to start a charity team, but the first blank—which asked for my team name—still had me stymied. *Team name? Team name? Team name?*

Nothing. I would have to come back to that.

I shot a quick text to Tom Kuhn, the medical assistant I worked with every day in my office. He liked to go by his initials: TK. I was sure that he would join the team, because TK sort of owed it to me. Not only had I chosen him, an applicant with *no* medical experience, to fill a position, but I had even convinced him to start running. I giggled to myself as I remembered those early years in my practice.

Suffice it to say, I am a difficult boss. Because I demand so much of myself, I accept no less from my employees. I hold everyone in my practice, from receptionist to biller to nurse, to the same exacting standard to which I hold myself. That standard is at times difficult for me to maintain, though, and therefore it is seemingly impossible for most of my medical assistants, who need to be compassionate, kind, funny, smart, on time, on the ball, and on task—sometimes on several tasks at once.

One winter in my first couple of years in practice, I hired Linda, an older, old-school Italian nurse with an impressive résumé. She had spent years on the cardiac unit of the hospital, where the sickest patients often were. Linda was meticulous in her appearance: short auburn hair sprayed into stiff wisps, red lipstick never venturing off her carefully lined mouth. Her unmistakable smoker's rasp greeted patients like old friends. Based on her life experience alone, she should have had no trouble keeping up in my office.

On one of Linda's first days, I came out of a patient room and said, "Mrs. S. is having palpitations and needs an ECG right now. After the ECG, she will need labs drawn for a CBC, CMP, TSH, T4, Ca, Mg, and Phos. How is Mr. R's pulmonary function? Make sure you walk him before that pulse ox. I will also need all of his discharge summaries from the hospital, and get his pulmonologist on the phone. Oh, and did I say Phos level for Mrs. S.?"

Linda was paralyzed. When she was finally able to move, she moved right out the front door and never came back. Needless to say, that happened several times. In fact, only a handful of nurses were able to handle the rigors of my practice and my neurotic tendencies while making it look easy.

Judy, my lead medical assistant, was ten years my senior. As a young girl, she was seriously burned when a pot of boiling water tipped over on her, and as an adult she would never be caught with her scarred arms, neck, or chest exposed. Her accident instilled in her a compassion that is impossible to teach and priceless in a medical practice. Judy also had a motherly ability to steer me in the right direction while remaining respectful to me. It did not take long for her to become my right-hand woman. She started with me on my very first day and has been with me since. Back in the early days, Judy did everything: took vitals, called patients, drew blood, and rearranged flowers, all the while waiting patiently for her first paycheck while my fledgling practice built up.

As the practice blossomed, she not only got paid but also got promoted over and over again. Eventually, her role became less about hands-on patient care and more about the behind-the-scenes tasks that kept our wheels turning. Judy soon took over my corner office, where she spent her days coordinating all aspects of patient care. She made urgent appointments with specialists, fetched needed results, and squeezed people into my overflowing schedule. Her voice became the voice of my practice. Patients would gently opt to speak to Judy over me. When Maisy was just five years old, she asked me to chaperone a school field trip. Disappointed that, as usual, I had to work, she said hopefully, "Hey, Mom! Can't you just ask Miss Judy if you can have a day off?"

After many failed medical assistants just like Linda, I hired TK to be my assistant. I met him first as a patient. He was my age and just needed a doctor. He was always tan and trim and had a smile that filled the room. TK heard that I was looking for an assistant and applied with an enthusiasm I had not encountered since Judy. When I hired him, he had no medical training at all, but he learned quickly. Like Judy's compassion, TK brought kindness to my practice. Patients quickly came to love his gentle way of giving a shot, his easy smile, and consoling manner.

TK became my work husband. Most weeks, I actually spent more time with him than I did with Chris. He met all of my requirements and was one of very few people allowed to tell me to "simmer down" when I got revved up. Our relationship seemed odd at first glance, yet it worked. He was always able to anticipate my needs, make my patients laugh, and, of critical importance, keep me moving from room to room without a hiccup.

Together, we also hatched a gingerbread-magnet scheme. The role of the magnet was simple: its presence would indicate which room I was needed in next. Before he ducked into a patient's room to complete a typically long list of tasks, TK would place the magnet on the door frame of the room I was to enter, just in case we missed each other. Now and again, I would use the magnet to hold little notes of instruction for TK. We took every opportunity to poke fun at each other with those notes and that magnet. A typical to-do list read:

1. ECG
2. Labs
3. Flu shot

TK would complete the tasks quietly and then hang a response note for me:

1. ~~ECG~~
2. ~~Labs~~
3. ~~Flu shot~~
4. F off

My staff took bets on how I would react upon noticing three gingerbread men stacked on top of each other in compromising positions. Once, around Christmastime, I blew into the room that our trusted magnet signal designated as my next in line, only to come face-to-face with a three-foot-tall Christmas tree decorated with speculums, tubes of lubricant, and garlands of rubber gloves. It became TK and Judy's mission to trip me—their seemingly unflappable boss—up.

Once, on a particularly hectic day, I stepped out of one room to take an urgent call. A few minutes later, I returned to the hallway to find four identical magnets on four patient doors. I stood crippled by indecision, before putting my hands up pleadingly. "Where to?" I questioned. The entire office staff erupted in laughter behind me, and I joined them.

The three of us made up a rock-star team. They understood me, and I was entirely dependent on them to do all I had to do. TK and I would move flawlessly through entire afternoons— sometimes seeing twenty or more patients—without ever speaking to each other. It was a dance beautifully choreographed by a cheap wooden magnet and the notes he held. Our jovial banter made the workdays easier and the spirit in the office lively.

Eventually, I convinced him to register for a 5K with me—a Memorial Day run honoring Delaney Farren, a three-year-old in the throes of what would become a five-year battle with leukemia. TK had never run a 5K before, so when he showed up on race day covered in all sorts of runner's paraphernalia, I openly laughed at him. Then, in an apologetic move, I put my arm around his broad shoulders and quietly vowed to sacrifice my own finish to help my friend and employee finish his first race ever. Unfortunately, it would be TK who demonstrated true runner's grit that day, crossing the finish line a full twenty-two seconds ahead of me.

For years, TK would take every opportunity to remind me of that twenty-two-second victory.

* * *

Sitting there at the computer on December 31, 2012, trying to come up with a name for our team, I laughed at myself. Back then, I was stunned TK had beat me at all. Today, TK could smoke me in a 5K, then go on to run a marathon afterward *and* make it look easy. He would be my first recruit. I knew a little throwdown with his "boss lady" would get his juices flowing.

"Hey, TK! How about a redo? Twenty-two secs on a 5K is nothin'! Let's do 10 miles! Broad Street, 5/5/13. You in?"

His instant reply launched our team. TK didn't realize it at the time, but in his response, he had also come up with our team name.

"Let's do it! CMMD, get ready to get your butt beat—again!"

He called me CMMD! Again, I laughed aloud recalling the ridiculousness of my new nickname. It had started a year before. In an effort to rebrand my medical practice, I had hired a graphic designer to create a logo for my practice. Leigh Friedman had magically transformed the name Christine Meyer, MD, into an immediately recognizable symbol: CMMD. The two *M*s were designed to look like people holding hands, symbolizing our doctor-patient partnerships. While the logo was an instant hit with patients and colleagues, it also served as instant fodder for my oft-insubordinate staff. They all insisted that while it was clever, it was also extremely narcissistic. They stopped calling me Christine, opting instead for CMMD. Phone messages would read, "CMMD, pls. call back." Sticky notes declared, "CMMD to review." Even the UPS driver would call, "Delivery for CMMD."

Months of playful teasing about my logo, coupled with TK's lazy texting, accidently named our Broad Street Run team: Team CMMD.

TK and I agreed that to really be considered legitimate, we needed at least a couple more people. My next text was to Joan, the family doctor who had joined my practice less than a year before.

* * *

By 2012, my practice had exploded in patient volume; between that and the acuity of ill patients like Debi, Joe, and Rosella, I quickly realized that I would need to hire a doctor to help decompress my schedule. The practice was clearly too big and too complex for me and my sole nurse-practitioner, Amy, to handle alone, so I put the word out that I was hiring.

Dr. Joan McFadden's e-mail inquiring about a job could not have been timed better. She had heard from a friend that I might be in the market to hire a physician, and she was moving back to the area from Massachusetts. "Maybe we should meet for coffee?" she asked.

Her CV was dazzling: she had attended the world-renowned University of Pennsylvania Medical School and completed her family-practice training at the University of Washington in Seattle. She was my age and had years of experience in primary care. Still, as I pored over her amazing credentials, I got an inexplicable feeling of melancholy. I was fully expecting to be disappointed—so much so that on that warm April Saturday morning of our prearranged meeting, I went for what would be one of my last long weekend runs before my involuntary running sabbatical. Not only did I not change my clothes, I did not even bother to shower before our meeting time.

I arrived twenty minutes early and sat alone by the door, analyzing every arriving Starbucks guest. All I knew about Joan was that she was my age and female. Every time the door opened, I studied face, posture, and clothing style. The first customers were too old, too young, too made-up, or too disheveled. As I sat there with my matted moist hair, flushed cheeks, and an unmistakable line of ass sweat shamelessly dampening my black running pants, I never once wondered how others, including my prospective employee, might see *me*.

The second Joan walked into the bustling coffee shop, there was no mistaking her. It was her eyebrows that first caught my attention. They were artfully shaped and meticulously groomed. Instinctively, I smoothed my own hopeless brows and kicked myself for not having bothered to shower. I would eventually figure out that I was obsessed with Joan's perfect brows because they demonstrated care, attention to detail, and mindfulness—all necessary attributes of a great doctor, and all things I was constantly striving to achieve. Sadly, that particular day, these attributes were not high on my list of things to put forward myself. Instead, I sat there squirming in my sweaty pants.

After talking with her for nearly two hours, I walked away utterly infatuated. Joan and I exchanged phone numbers and promised to call each other. As we turned our separate ways, I noticed her legs. The simple sundress she wore modestly brushed the tops of her knees. She was thin but not frail. In fact, her muscular calves had me eying my own capri pants with a bit of self-loathing as images of elephants raced through my mind. One thing was painfully clear to me: I had to have her.

I wasn't yet home when I dialed her number from my cell to tell her that I *really* liked her and that I was *really* hoping we could work out the business stuff *really* fast. She had an easy, comfortable laugh that told me we would get along just fine.

That night, I read Joan's CV for the ninth time. The last section detailed her hobbies, which we had not gotten a chance to talk about. When she "was not hard at work," Joan loved to "ski and compete in sprint triathlons."

What? She's a runner! I knew it was meant to be.

An hour later, I had carefully crafted an e-mail offering Joan the job. I ended it with "By the way, you run? I run! Hey, what's a sprint triathlon?"

In the few days it took for her to respond, I replayed that last line over and over again in my mind.

"What's a sprint triathlon?" Seriously? Why would you ask her that? She's probably thinking you're a computer illiterate who's never Googled anything before. And, why, why, why would you call yourself a runner? Did you see her legs? You, my friend, are no runner—you don't deserve her.

In true fairy-tale style, and just when I had convinced myself I had driven her away, Joan finally responded to my e-mail and graciously accepted my job offer.

Not only was she a great doctor and a great addition to my practice, Joan was also searingly competitive. Within hours of learning of Team CMMD's inception, she signed on as our third runner, loudly declaring that she would happily run TK into the ground.

Clare-E Nanacassee was my third recruit. She was a gifted baker, a serious runner, and one of my most vivid lessons in forgiveness. Her real name was Clare Elizabeth, but she had decided to refer to herself as Clare-E—"it just feels right," she explained. Years before she became Team CMMD's fourth runner, Clare-E had worked for me as a medical assistant. She was great with patients, smart, and dedicated. She also had an inexplicable obsession with her weight that powered her around the streets of Downingtown at all hours of the day and night. She ran hundreds of miles in an openly displayed effort to "get skinny." Despite the abuse her hands took as a skilled pastry chef and artist, as a medical assistant, she had the gentlest of touches. Men insisted on having her administer their testosterone shots. They all had the same dreamy smile as they explained, "I don't know how she does it, but when Clare-E gives me that shot, I barely feel it."

Then one day, she quit abruptly. The bakery she worked for had promised her a partnership she could not turn down.

I knew Clare-E would be impossible to replace, so I was not gracious about her leaving and did not wish her well. In fact, one day after her resignation, I asked her to pack her things and leave. Although I knew full well that I still needed her help, I tersely told her that her services were no longer necessary. Within twenty-four hours, I had terminated her from our payroll, paying her for the two weeks' notice I had turned down. I took back her office key and even unfriended her on Facebook.

TK and others in my office apparently saw the irrationality of my vengeful move long before I did. Two years later, as Joan was getting ready to start, Judy, the lead nurse and patient care coordinator who had helped me build my practice, cornered me and began, "Christine, with Joan starting, we need another nurse. TK and I just cannot run all three of you like this."

I nodded. I had seen this coming. Everyone was spread thin.

TK blurted out, "We want you to hire Clare-E back. The bakery let her go, and she *needs* this job. You know she's great. We will never find anyone like her."

My face flushed and my heart pounded. *"No. Way."*

Judy's voice was even. "We know she left us in the lurch, but that was two years ago. She had to make the best decision for her family. They promised her a million-dollar business! How could she say no? Why are you being so irrational about this?"

At home that evening, I flopped on my bed, fully dressed, and unloaded the whole sordid story on Chris. "I'm just so mad that she left! I know it's totally irrational; I just can't get over that."

He picked my legs up and laid them on his lap. As he rubbed my feet, he asked, "Why did she leave in the first place?"

"Because she had a potentially great opportunity for her family." I was exasperated. It was a stupid question to which he knew the answer.

"Can you really blame her? If you were offered a once-in-a-lifetime opportunity to better yourself, wouldn't you take it?" he asked quietly.

As he got up, he called over his shoulder, "You would. Don't be stubborn—you're just spiting yourself now."

I stomped around my bedroom for a few minutes, annoyed that he had called me out *again* but knowing he was right.

* * *

The next week, Clare-E arrived for our second "interview" dressed in torn jeans and sporting a new radical haircut and nose ring. Clare-E's edginess and grunge would seem out of place in my meticulously designed and professionally decorated medical office. But, like that last squirt of lime on a piece of cooked fish, Clare-E brought a zing and freshness that I craved.

It was only when she began to speak that it occurred to me that she was nervous.

"I-I want you to know how much this job means to me." Her mouth was dry, and she instinctively reached for the massive bottle of water she always seemed to carry.

"Don't let me down." The gruff words barely suppressed the smile that was just beginning to curl the corners of my mouth.

The real reason I couldn't turn Clare-E away was that she was good. In fact, when it came to patient care and advocacy, Clare-E was great. She had an inherent ability to put herself in a patient's position. After her first few months on the job, years before, not only had Clare-E mastered the painless injection technique that left people asking for her by name, but when bad weather threatened to keep older patients from their appointments, she had offered to drive them to and from the office. She had a kind heart and a gentle touch—and no matter how hard I tried to ignore those traits, I knew she was an essential addition to my staff.

About a month after she started working for me again, Clare-E brought me a small bud vase of baby roses. The handwritten note said, "Thanks for everything. Here's to second chances and many more years. Love, Clare-E"

Now, Clare-E's response to my short text asking her to join

the rest of Team CMMD as we ran the Philadelphia Broad Street Run was simple: "Wouldn't miss it!" She went on to say that since she ran all the time anyway and was downright terrified of letting me down ever again, she would happily join us.

Once we had our team of four in place, I started a Team CMMD Runs Broad Street Facebook page and invited all my friends and fans to like it. The total calculated reach was in the tens of thousands. We all shamelessly harangued every runner we could think of to join the team.

I had been openly telling my aunt's story to raise awareness for colon cancer screening. Clare-E had lost her forty-six-year-old cousin, Ritaanne, to metastatic melanoma. Much like Debi McLaughlin, Ritaanne had been a vibrant young mother. In addition to Debi's five young children, this ruthless disease had orphaned Ritaanne's two children when they were both younger than five. TK was running for his older brother, Glenn, who, like Ritaanne and Debi, had died in his early forties. His was an aggressive tongue cancer that took too long to diagnose, and he died just ten months later.

As the four of us took to social media to share these devastating tales and our intentions to run Broad Street "for those who couldn't run for themselves," we posted long narratives on each of our personal fundraising pages, Facebook, and Twitter. We pasted flyers around the office and made gigantic posters inviting people to support our team. Over the next few months, we all talked to friends, family, patients, and business owners about making a donation or, better yet, joining Team CMMD.

Like metal shavings drawn to a magnet, people of all and no running abilities signed up. Many had heard of Broad Street and wanted the chance to run without worrying about the lottery to participate. Many were patients and knew all of us through my practice. Many had weight to lose or shape to regain. And practically all had a heartbreaking cancer story to share.

Chapter 5: A Rivalry Is Born

Rivalry isn't hate; it is a partnership in disguise.

—Anonymous

Tom O'Grady, Amy's husband, had not been in my house more than ten minutes when he began lifting lids and sticking his nose into every bowl and pot on my counter. I had only just met the man, and there he stood, invading my most sacred of spaces: the kitchen. *My* kitchen.

In late 2007, shortly after Hadley was born, I had decided to hire a nurse-practitioner to help me manage my growing practice. Amy O'Grady was kind, smart, and well trained. I offered and she accepted, neither of us with hesitation. Shortly after it became "official," I invited the O'Gradys over for dinner. I hoped that our families could get to know each other while enjoying a homemade meal. As I finished up my prep, I was smug. In my mind, this supper of seared chicken breasts, my aunt's *rozz*, and homemade tortilla chips with fresh mango salsa was simple and delicious.

Tom O. was a big, confident man. Like Chris, he kept his short beard neatly trimmed but had chosen to shave his head completely. I had always been intimidated by bald, confident men, and Tom O.'s reluctant smile only deepened my nervousness in his presence. He was the kind of man who just took over a room. He loved to talk about hunting deer and turkey. Years later, as I watched him cook, I would wonder how those murderous hands could one day tear open an animal's belly to pull out viscera and the next create something beautiful and delicate in the kitchen.

There he stood, snooping around my pots and pans with the same intrusiveness as a guest snooping around a bathroom medicine cabinet. As he started dipping spoons and tasting, I stepped back and donned my best humble, *who, me?* smile. Then I stood aside, waiting for the barrage of accolades that he, like nearly everyone else who had ever tasted my cooking, would shower upon me. I braced myself for the dreamy, stunned look he was bound to get the second my homemade mango salsa touched his lips. It was amazing—a little sweet and a little spicy, with a palate-cleansing freshness that finely grated lime zest imparted.

I tried my best to read Tom O.'s face, but it was like stone. He made no indication to me whether he loved my salsa or hated it.

Now, I have an undeniable obsession with food. I read food magazines and watch food shows. I buy cookbooks for beach reading and consider food shopping a hobby. This food obsession has everything to do with my extended Egyptian family, especially Tant. Not only was her pot of *rozz* ever present and always delicious, but it was usually only one of six or seven dishes on her typical weeknight dinner table. On any cold, wet night, I found myself craving her *molokhia bil rozz*, a peasant soup classically served over rice.

To Egyptians, making *molokhia* (pronounced *mow-low-kheeya*) is a painstaking process steeped in tradition. It begins by finely chopping the coarse leaves of this herbaceous green vegetable, which are similar in shape to mint leaves but at least twice as large. *Molokhia* is indigenous to Egypt, where the balmy climate and fertile Nile delta provide an ideal growing environment. There exists absolutely no comparable flavor.

Once the large *molokhia* leaves were plucked off the stems, they were washed, carefully dried, and piled into a huge mound on layers of newspaper. Chopping them was often my grandmother's job. Tayta sat at the table, gripping both handles of the *makhrata*, a large, curved kitchen tool whose only purpose was to chop *molokhia* leaves. Two wooden grips held the razor-sharp blade in place. Keeping her elbows tucked in, and with the smallest motion of her wrists, Tayta rocked the blade through the pile of leaves in a mowing motion. After every pass, she scraped and gathered the chopped leaves back to the middle of the soggy newspaper. Chop. Scrape. Gather. Chop. Scrape. Gather. My grandmother repeated the process until the mountain of *molokhia* leaves was reduced to a small mound of thick paste. My aunt and grandmother could tear through twenty cups of leaves in fifteen minutes, but an inexperienced cook might spend hours getting the consistency just right.

Then Tayta pinched a bit of the *molokhia* paste and rubbed her thumb and forefinger together. Once she was satisfied with the texture, she would slide the green mound into a rich home-made chicken stock that had been simmering on the stove for hours. As the pulverized leaves released their proteins, the soup took on a gelatinous thickness and bright green color. Despite the arduous process from leaves to paste to soup, the final and defining layer of *molokhia*'s distinctive flavor took just seconds to achieve. Making *tasha*, chopped garlic fried in butter or lard, was the last critical step in the making of *molokhia*. *Tasha* took a young girl years to master and—along with wide, sturdy hips—made her a most desirable bride.

The Arabic word *tasha* comes from the sizzling sound of hot, bubbling grease mixing dangerously with liquid. A pot of *molokhia* can be made or broken by the quality of that *tasha*. After setting the *molokhia* to simmer, Tayta would turn her attention to an entire head of garlic, sometimes more. This time, her tool was a large wooden mortar and pestle. Her meticulous rocking was replaced by a rhythmic pounding that reduced the mountain of pearly cloves to a tablespoon or two of pungent garlic paste.

Tayta was also serious about butter—only the real deal would suffice for browning the garlic paste. With the butter still foaming, my grandmother would, in one motion, pluck the entire red-hot metal skillet—garlic, butter, and all—off its burner and dunk it fully into the simmering pot of *molokhia*. The unmistakable sound and rich garlic scent was all we ever needed to race down to my aunt's overflowing table.

When I was about eleven or twelve, my father got the idea to try to grow *molokhia* in our backyard. The cool New Jersey climate and sandy, soil of the Pine Barrens were about as far from what all believed to be the absolute necessities for a good crop. Everyone thought he was nuts for trying. However, not only did my father achieve a delicious and bountiful crop that year, but he also figured out that the chopped leaves could be flash frozen, cutting *molokhia*'s prep time dramatically.

Growing up, I loved *molokhia* the way some kids love lima beans: passionately, but with a bit of peer-induced shame. I quickly learned to be ashamed of my favorite Egyptian foods as they made appearances in my school lunches. Opening a thermos of *molokhia* in third grade had about the same effect on American kids as throwing up right on the table. Countless times, I put on my pathetic face as lunchtime approached. My teachers would shake their heads and send me to the office for my "free cheese sandwich" voucher. It never occurred to me that some janitor was finding a thermos full of garlicky, mucusy-green substance in the bathroom garbage about once a week.

When my mother could no longer afford to replace my thermoses, she packed me fava bean sandwiches in pita bread. Those, too, routinely found their way into the girls' lavatory wastebasket. Years later, in my saddest times, I would close my eyes and imagine those half rounds of bread stuffed with a creamy fava bean mixture and fresh cucumbers, or that thick, garlicky soup that used to warm my soul from the inside out. Invariably, these daydreams led me to the kitchen, where I would concoct new recipes—ones that often had nothing to do with the Egyptian food I started out craving. My famous mango salsa was created in that very way.

* * *

Tom's eyes did widen a bit as he crunched one of my just-out-of-the-fryer chips. He savored the tiny bit of meticulously chopped salsa the way some savored wine. I instantly recognized the de-liberation his palate was making. Then, instead of showering compliments, he said, "Hey, did you ever think about putting fresh cilantro in that?"

What?

Here was this guy whom I had known for only moments, whose wife I had granted the privilege of working for me, who had just sniffed and poked his way around in *my* space, and he was giving *me* cooking tips?

The worst thing for me was that he was completely right. My fridge and pantry were never without an array of spices and herbs, and that night was no exception. I offered him a bunch of cilantro with the formality of someone extending an olive branch. Tom O. was left-handed, and I immediately picked up on his two-second pause as I handed him my world-class *santoku* chef's knife. With an expert hand, he made quick work of the cilantro and sprinkled it onto my bowl of nearly superb salsa with a flourish. The cilantro Tom O. added to that mixture brought it to life. Moreover, his ability to deliver an unabridged critique of my cooking made him an instant and lifelong friend.

The night we first met, Tom O. and I learned a few things about each other. First, we were both hopeless food nerds and could watch *Iron Chef* 24-7. Second, we both dreamed in copper pots and hand-forged German knives. I'm not sure which one of us leaped up more quickly as Chris tried to put that *santoku* into the dishwasher—he might as well have been about to drop a baby onto the tile floor. Lastly, after a night of bickering over things like blond versus brown roux and whether to brine or not to brine a turkey, it became obvious to all that he and I were both fiercely competitive. It was the night we met that the Meyer-O'Grady kitchen rivalry was born.

* * *

Turning our love of food and that intense but amiable rivalry into an evening of entertainment for our friends came naturally. Our first cook-off was simple and decided by a "show of hands." Tom O. took that one home on the back of the most succulent ribs I had ever tasted. Our next competition was in a class of its own. Our guests ate for three hours while marking scorecards that I had created on my home computer. That landslide and hand-hammered copper risotto pot were all mine, although Tom O. bemoaned the biased audience, as most of the guests that night were my friends. "The next cook-off will be a totally blind tiebreaker," he vowed.

Tom O. and I turned these cook-offs into a tradition over the next five years, so by the time Team CMMD had taken shape and we had committed to trying to raise a significant amount of money for the American Cancer Society, he and I knew exactly what our main fund-raising event would be. Tom O. was not a runner, but his own dear aunt Kathy, my patient, had died of lung cancer just days after I started the team. He, like I, had a guttural need to do something big to support all those battling cancer—and of course it would involve food.

By mid-January, just two weeks after its inception, Team CMMD had over twenty runners. While the donations trickled in, we began planning the competition in earnest. Tom O. and I vowed that we would carry out this contest in epic style to honor both of our aunts.

The idea was simple enough. We would follow the same basic principles of our last contest but do so on a much larger scale. Instead of feeding our friends for bragging rights, we would charge admission and hold a silent auction during the dinner to raise money for our cause. On Thursday night, January 18, 2013, I posted on the team's Facebook page, asking any members interested in helping with our main event to come to a brainstorming session the next weekend.

That night, I did not sleep well. I was overwhelmed and unsure of the cohesiveness of our team. The fact that we had now enrolled more than twenty runners meant we needed to raise a minimum of $10,000 collectively to ensure a race bib for everyone on the team. As of that Thursday afternoon, we had raised about $7,000.

As was my routine, the next morning at 5:30, I sat with my coffee and logged on to our team page, which was set up to prominently display our team's fund-raising total in the top right corner. No matter what else was happening on that page, my eyes gravitated to that corner first.

I blinked to clear what I was sure was sleepy blurriness from my eyes. There was no mistake. In just under nine hours, our team total had jumped by over $2,000. Until that moment, the dollars had trickled in slowly in increments of $20, $30, or $100. I had never seen such a huge increase in such a short time.

I had to know which runners had scored these big donations. As team captain, I was able to view the roster and could tell how much each runner had raised individually. A quick look at the team stats revealed that one person had donated all $2,000, and to *me*—Kristy Harper.

Kristy was a good friend and running buddy. She had signed on to the team practically the moment I asked her to. She was just "good people." She and her husband, Brock, owned a wildly successful physical therapy practice in our town, and they were as dedicated to their patients as I was to mine. Kristy's quiet, unsolicited donation was exactly in keeping with the unassuming way she lived her life. Despite working harder than anyone I knew and reaping just financial rewards, she kept her lifestyle simple and modest.

As I digested the implications of that donation, I began to cry. With that single gesture, Kristy had sponsored four runners who might not otherwise have made their minimum.

I had to speak to my friend to thank her personally. After leaving messages at all of her numbers, I recorded a video on my computer, though I was still in my pajamas, unshowered, and not wearing an ounce of makeup. As the camera on my Mac recorded, I described my young team and my aunt's story, which had started it all. I told of our progress to date and then gave a tearful description of Kristy's heart-stopping donation. Without a moment's hesitation, I posted the video on every social media outlet I was connected to.

Kristy's donation and my thank-you video started an unbelievable rally. By the end of that day, our team had raised nearly $11,000. Donations poured in, along with comments like *Thank you so much for starting this team*, and *Dr. M., I don't know you or your dear friend Kristy, but that video made me fall in love with you both*. That last, anonymous comment came with a donation of $250. And as the dollars streamed in, so did runners. It seemed as if everyone who learned of us wanted to be a part of our effort.

Emboldened by Kristy's donation, I issued a challenge to my team to raise our collective fund-raising goal to $20,000, which meant we would have to raise nearly $10,000 more. The cook-off and silent auction would need to be a huge success if we had any chance of meeting our new objective.

Only a handful of people showed up to our event planning meeting that weekend. As I sat and looked at the few volunteers who were there, my heart sank. There was just no way we would pull off an event of the scale we needed to with so few people. Tom O. would not be deterred, however. "We can totally do it!" he insisted. His confidence did little to assuage me, but I went along, feeling like I really had no choice and hoping that the power of his certainty would create some magical force to draw volunteers.

Our first order of business was to choose the date. Saturday, February 23, 2013, seemed ideal for several reasons. First, it was a midway point between the date of our team's creation and the May 5 race day. Second, it would be a miserable, dreary, postholidays time of year. We were sure people would be eager for something fun to do. The only problem with that date was that it gave us just under five weeks to pull the whole thing off. We needed a strategy, a place, a budget, and a marketing plan—and we needed all those things in a hurry. Then Tom O. and I would really have our work cut out for us. We, two home cooks who had cooked only for household dinner parties, would have to figure out how to make enough food for that many people—especially given the style of the dinner we wanted to present.

That night, we all talked about what we were trying to do for this charity and for cancer sufferers. To all of us at the meeting, the word "fight" came naturally. Our patients and loved ones were fighting their diseases, people said they were in for the "fight" of their lives, and the rivalry Tom O. and I had lent itself nicely to the whimsical concept of a "food fight." We were going to use food as a weapon in our collective battle against this hateful disease.

Leigh, the graphic designer who had created the now-well-known CMMD logo, would design shirts, programs, and voting cards. She introduced me to her friend TJ, who would make a great emcee. TJ's wife, Maria, had been a regular supporter of the American Cancer Society and was eager to help in any way she could.

Tom O. and I had a very clear vision of how the night would play out, even though everyone at the meeting, including our spouses, shook their heads. No one believed we could pull off such an elaborate scheme. Our plan was to serve two five-course meals to at least one hundred seated and paying guests. Each chef would be required to prepare an appetizer, soup, salad, an entrée, and dessert. The dishes would be presented one at a time and without any hint to our guests as to which chef had prepared what. With every course, scorecards would be distributed, describing the dishes about to be served. After savoring the tasting portions of each course, the guests would score each plate on three criteria: taste, originality, and plating. At the conclusion of every course, the cards would be collected and the scores tallied, and when the night ended, the chef with the highest score would be named the winner.

Once we had worked out the structure and rough plan of the night, we had to get down to the details. We knew our food fight was happening; we just didn't know where—and without a location, none of the rest of that elaborate plan mattered. The venue had to be large enough to seat one hundred guests. It also had to be local and have a fully equipped restaurant kitchen. But perhaps the most daunting requirement was that its owner had to be willing to loan the restaurant to a bunch of amateurs for one night in exchange for little or no compensation. To rent a location would cut heavily into our funds for the charity, so we needed to keep all of our costs as low as possible.

Patti and Pauly Frank came to all of our minds immediately. They were an adorable couple from Louisiana who owned the Blue Cafe. Their little restaurant was smack in the middle of our small town. Pauly was famous for his breakfast and lunch creations but had vowed never to do a dinner service. "After two P.M., I just wanna live my life," he often drawled in explanation.

As we talked it over, the room fell silent. Who would be brave enough to ask the Franks for such an enormous favor? All eyes turned to me.

"What? Why me?" I asked, with an unmistakable whine.

"You're their doctor!" Tom O. said. "They have to say yes to you!"

I couldn't argue. Patti and Pauly's place was a no-brainer, especially since they didn't serve dinner, so our takeover of their space for an evening would not necessarily be a huge imposition. In return, we could offer to shamelessly promote their business at every opportunity. "We will leave your place cleaner than we find it!" I promised in the e-mail I sent before our meeting had even adjourned. In a tone just shy of begging, I described my aunt, Tom O.'s aunt, our team, and the crazy idea for the food fight. Then we all held our breath.

Because we had so little time until our date, we could not wait for the Franks' polite refusal to look at other options. Our plan B needed to be in the works before we even heard from them. Our best bet turned out to be a local banquet hall that had a kitchen and a large, open room and was available that night for $800.

Finally, we had a glimmer of hope. While that was more money than we wanted to spend, we still hadn't heard from Patti and Pauly and felt as if we had no choice. I asked the manager to send a contract to me that day, but within moments, my heart sank. "There's just one thing," she said, with an unmistakable smoker's rasp. "If you and your friend are going to do all the cooking, you have to have a food handler's license—health department rules." She did not care that I was a physician and had a license that allowed me to handle life-and-death situations. It was a food handler's license or bust. A few phone calls later, and I learned that it would take at least four to six weeks to get that government-issued document—meaning, it would be impossible.

In desperation, I did what had worked for me all along in this process: I posted a plea on Facebook for someone with a food handler's license willing to work the kitchen with Tom O. and me that night.

No more than an hour later, Loretta Parks messaged me: "I have a food handler's license! And by the way, I do a lot of charity baking, so I know a few things about cooking for crowds and raising money!"

Relief washed over me as I pulled the banquet agreement off my home fax machine. I planned on dropping it off, along with a check, at the hall the next morning.

It turned out we never had to use Loretta's license or my check for $800 after all. That evening, I got a simply worded e-mail response from the Franks. "We would love to help! Just tell us what and when."

Saturday, February 23, 2013, was open for the Blue Cafe. Fortunately, their bustling catering side business did not have a commitment that night. Within seconds of receiving Patti's e-mail, I sent a barrage of all-caps texts to nearly a dozen people. "THEY SAID YES! FOOD FIGHT 2013 IS A GO!"

Like a theater troupe of understudies who had rehearsed together a hundred times and were praying for a chance to perform, we all sprang into action. Everyone knew what they had to do. I created a free Eventbrite site, which allowed me to collect money and sell tickets electronically. We already had great photos of Tom O. and me wielding furious faces and sharp knives. Now that our place and date were set, we simply needed to print the posters. We added a QR code to each one so that, with the click of a button from any smartphone, people could purchase tickets from anywhere at any time.

Pauly Frank had said that we could easily seat eighty to one hundred guests in his restaurant. "But remember," he warned, "y'all gotta cook for all those people!" He smiled knowingly as Tom O. and I shrugged our shoulders in blissful naïveté. "And I got four walls for ya, plus a kitchen, a fridge, a pantry, and even some dishes, but I *don't* have a staff—unless y'all wanna pay 'em."

No. We did not want to pay a staff. We would need to get volunteers to do everything from setting up to serving to cleaning up.

Our ticket prices seemed hefty at $75 per individual or $125 per couple, but Tom O. had convinced me that for ten restaurant-quality plates of food per person, that was a steal. "Plus," he pointed out, "people are going to be entertained for an *entire* night—watching me kick their beloved Dr. Meyer's ass in the kitchen!"

So began thirty-four days of frenetic planning, complete with daily smack talk and subterfuge plotting, for Tom O. and me. We completed our poster with a slogan that was an absolute reflection of Leigh's talent.

2 CHEFS

5 COURSES

10 PLATES

1 MISSION: TO HELP LOVED ONES AND STRANGERS
AS THEY FIGHT FOR THEIR LIVES

We planned to hang a life-size poster advertising the upcoming event in the Blue Cafe, in hopes of attracting some of the Franks' regulars. I had extra takeaway flyers printed to stack around my office. We prayed that we could sell enough tickets to justify the amount of work this event would take. Meanwhile, Amy volunteered to commandeer the silent-auction half of the event. For her second in command, she recruited Karen Baker.

Karen was a thirty-eight-year-old patient of mine with twin ten-year-old girls. She had been diagnosed with a rare and aggressive sarcoma of the thigh two years before. In the time since her diagnosis, she had had five surgeries, endured both chemo and radiation, and dealt with chronic pain and near-daily fear that her cancer would recur or metastasize. Not only did Karen hobble all over town on her bad leg, trying to secure donations and sponsorships, but on one sleeting, gray afternoon she was forced to endure a tongue lashing from a local pub owner.

In response to her earnest plea on behalf of our team, the owner of a popular family eatery loosed on Karen his beliefs about the "real story" behind cancer in this country. He explained how cancer was really a fabrication of our government as it sought to elevate its image by finding "cures" for diseases that really did not exist. He went on to tell her that people would not get cancer if they simply lived cleaner, healthier lives. "What do people think is going to happen if they keep smoking, drinking, and eating like pigs?" he cried.

Without missing a beat, Karen thanked him for his time and asked him when we all might expect his new pub menu: one devoid of fried, greasy food and beer. After all, he didn't want to contribute to the cancer epidemic, did he? As strong as she was in her face-to-face confrontation, Karen's voice shook on the phone as she recounted the dreadful conversation to me. She felt utterly humiliated as she hobbled out on her throbbing leg—empty-handed.

I was furious, but I knew that I could not verbally destroy this man or his local business, as such an action would reflect poorly on our team and the positive impact we had had on our community in just four weeks. Instead, I logged on to my practice Facebook page and summarized Karen's story, taking care not to mention any identifiable details of that restaurant or its wifty owner.

Supporters of our team were as outraged as I was and rallied behind Karen and her efforts on our behalf. Dozens of commentators begged me to share the name of the restaurant so they could boycott it and its owner. In the end, despite the fact that I kept the identity of that business between Karen and me, two amazing things happened. First, our team donations skyrocketed. In the hours after that post, we raised an additional $2,500, which brought our team total to nearly $16,000. Second, I was able to secure the most important member of my food fight team. Karen's husband, James, signed on as my sous chef. He, too, was a Food Network junkie, had a few tricks up his sleeve, and had to do something worthwhile for our cause and, by extension, for his wife—a cancer warrior herself.

By February 1, 2013, Tom O. and I had assembled our kitchen teams. Loretta, our licensed food handler; Karen's husband, James; and another food nerd–patient, named Arlen, rounded out my team. Tom O. had quickly claimed Clare-E, my nurse and master baker. With her, Tom O. had a definite edge, as she was also an accomplished artist. Since presentation was one of the three categories we would be judged on, I was certain Tom O. would put Clare-E in charge of plating. Clare-E's husband, Mala, naturally complemented her; since he worked the line at Applebee's, he had plenty of experience in the inner workings of a restaurant kitchen.

The last pair of hands on Tom O.'s formidable team belonged to Jack Schmidt. Not only was Jack a testicular-cancer survivor, but his wife had been diagnosed with sarcoma while he was still undergoing treatment for his own illness. Despite their simultaneous cancer battle, the Schmidts were really emotionally invested in this charity for their son, Thomas, who was just seven years old when he, like his mother, was diagnosed with a soft-tissue sarcoma. In the midst of our food fight preparation, Thomas was recovering from surgery to remove the cancerous growth from his leg.

I had not really understood how Jack found the strength to work so hard for our cause, even as his little boy lay in a hospital bed, until I asked him, "Jack, what are you doing here?"

Jack had arrived at one of many team meetings to discuss the details of the event. "Sitting in that hospital room next to him does not help Thomas at all. Being here, raising money for research, supporting so many who have it worse than we do . . . now, that's actually *doing* something for my Thomas."

* * *

We sold one hundred tickets to the food fight within three days of confirming our venue and finalizing the date. We even started a waiting list. Friends, family, patients, and even complete strangers were clamoring for tickets. We visited with Pauly one morning exactly thirty days from the team's inception. He and Patti were finishing up a typical busy breakfast service. Tom O. and I walked the restaurant and counted every nook and cranny we might be able to squeeze guests into. We could seat not one more than 104 people.

One of the two couples we called up off the waiting list offered to buy four more tickets. "Oh, I am so sorry," I explained, "but we are totally sold out—we can't squeeze any more people into our space."

The woman was kind. "Oh, honey! We're not *all* going to come. I just want to buy the extra tickets as a donation to the team."

It seemed as if, over the last month, I had been moved to tears at least once per day. This latest, $375 donation left me scrambling to maintain my composure yet again.

A quick look at the Eventbrite site for the food fight showed us that we had already collected over $6,000 in ticket money. While we would need to take out overhead expenses, many of the silent-auction items Karen and Amy were securing were nothing short of extravagant. Countless golf foursomes to prestigious local courses would bring several hundred dollars each. The owner of a local furniture shop that sold one-of-a-kind pieces made by Amish craftsmen offered up a large pie cupboard that retailed for $600. In my mind, I tallied the donations in the hundreds of dollars with satisfaction as all the smaller parts became an undeniable sum.

On a bitterly cold Tuesday afternoon, I took a call from Amy. She could barely hide the excitement in her voice.

"We just got a weekend in Canada!"

"What are you talking about?" Sleeplessness and stress were getting the better of me, and I did not have the patience to decipher her cryptic sentence.

"Christine! A couple just donated a weekend stay in their Niagara Falls vineyard! We could get *thousands* for that!"

That was the moment in which the magnitude of the money we were raising sank in. One event, one of many auction items, thousands of dollars. That Niagara Falls stay alone could fund two colonoscopies or twenty mammograms. We were actually going to make a tangible difference in the cancer fight.

I hung up with Amy and, for what seemed like the hundredth time, buried my face in my hands and cried.

With every passing day and every secured auction item, I had less doubt that by the time the last dish was washed, we would be able to exceed our goal of raising a total of $20,000 for the American Cancer Society. We had never dreamed that two home cooks serving over one thousand plates of restaurant-quality food would net over $9,000 in profits, much less transform a roster of forty strangers with only a love of running in common into a band of true friends for life.

Rules were agreed upon and teams finalized; tickets were sold and auction items procured. Tom O. and I worked out our menus and recipes and made lists of necessary dishes, silverware, and glasses. With less than three weeks till the food fight, we just had to figure out how in the world we were going to cook all that food, serve it quickly to over one hundred people, and time it so that every guest could browse our auction items without ever feeling like they were waiting for the next dish. We certainly didn't have the answers all worked out, but we were sure of one thing: we were going to need a lot of help.

Chapter 6: No Cake. No Spinach.

Tell me what you eat, and I will tell you who you are.

—Jean Anthelme Brillat-Savarin

Chris looked deflated as I set the small bowl in front of him. It was the eighth time in three weeks that I had forced him to eat my braised short ribs. I was living, breathing, and sleeping this food fight, and my family was along for the ride. As soon as our 104 tickets had sold out, I had begun creating a menu and building recipes. One of the most important rules of our contest was that all of our dishes had to be original, not re-created from another recipe or copied from a celebrity chef. Five courses meant five recipes to write, practice, and fine-tune. Almost since its inception, the food fight had been one of the most anticipated events in our community, and it had to live up to the hype.

But for me, pulling off the massive task, raising money for the American Cancer Society, and serving our guests not one, but two, perfect meals were secondary goals. I needed to *win* this contest. I needed to win for Tant, Rosella, Debi, and Joe. I needed to be good at something again.

The Egyptian food of my childhood is simple and rustic. *Rozz* and *molokhia* are created with more soul than science; family recipes are handed down without mention of measurements, temperatures, and cooking times. Egyptian women like Tant seem to have a cooking instinct that renders the need for those guidelines obsolete.

When I was in middle school, I had to complete an assignment to prepare an authentic Egyptian dish, provide the recipe, and demonstrate how the dish was made. My teacher was forced to give me a C for the project. "I'm sorry," she wrote on my paper. "A coffee cup is *not* a one-cup measure and 'kinda like this' is not a proper instruction. The stuffed grape leaves were delicious, however!"

At home, I cooked with that same instinct, but for this contest, I needed to channel my innermost scientist, mathematician, and engineer. My food fight meal had to be painstakingly planned, from recipe to prep to execution to plating. I could leave nothing to chance.

While I wasn't exactly sure *what* I was going to make, I was certain of a few facts. First, I would absolutely not make anything that night that I'd never made before. Second, my dishes would be sophisticated in flavor profile and plating but relatively simple to put together. I had to be able to do as many things ahead of time as possible. My team and I were going to serve 520 plates of food in a three-hour period. Meticulous planning and maximum efficiency would be critical to pulling off this massive event.

Chris didn't have quite the same enthusiasm for my eighth rib trial as he had for the first, but he smiled at me. I must have been a sight that dreary Sunday afternoon. My hair was a frazzled mess piled high on my head. Splotches of sauce dotted my apron, pants, and right cheek. My kitchen had been in a state of destruction for days, as I cooked, tested, and forced Chris to taste. During those weeks, I would come home from work, pull out my massive notebook, put an apron on over my work clothes, and get down to business. The first nights were great, because we had better weeknight dinners than ever, but by now, Chris and the kids were developing "taster fatigue."

In our marriage, one thing was a given: I cooked, and Chris cleaned up after me. Yet even during these crazy weeks leading up to the food fight, even as he washed and scrubbed and dried, only to repeat the same ritual night after night, his tone never got edgy. In fact, with every dishwasher load he emptied, he seemed to brighten.

Something about the way Chris was looking at me that Sunday afternoon of the rib trial made me pause. "What? Don't you like it? Too much soy sauce? Last time better? No. It was the third one—the one with twice the soy and half the tomato. That was the best, wasn't it?" As I rambled, I smoothed my dirty apron nervously over my thigh and blew a rogue curl off my face.

Chris put down his fork and walked over to me. As he tucked the stubborn curl behind my ear, he said, "No. I don't know which short ribs were the best. All I know is that seeing you pattering around the kitchen again gives me peace. If I have to eat short ribs every day for the rest of my life to see *that* smile, so be it. And, just so you know, these are the worst ones yet— you're overthinking it." With that, he kissed my cheek, shrugged on his coat, and headed out.

While I didn't necessarily agree with him that that last trial of short ribs was "the worst yet," he was right about everything else. Almost immediately after Team CMMD was created, something inside me changed. I felt excited, joyful, and happy. For the first time in months, I looked forward to things. The positive energy at home and in the office was palpable and came out in many different ways.

Weeks earlier, on a particularly crazy Monday in the office, right in the middle of patient hours, a cheer suddenly erupted from our front desk. TK had just logged on to the team page to see that our fund-raising total was just $235 shy of the $10,000 mark. Without wasting a second, I issued a challenge to my team. "All we need is for each of us to raise $5 to hit the $10,000 mark. Can we do it in the next hour?" As would become habitual for my team, not only did they welcome my challenge, they doubled the amount I asked for. It was like a bag of microwave popcorn—the first popped kernel set off an explosion. As soon as one person posted a plea on Facebook, the next one went, and so on and so on. The speed with which these things happened for our team, from raising money to selling tickets to securing silent-auction donations, was attributable to the power of two factors: the spirit of people truly committed to a cause, and the reach of social media.

At home, the air seemed to be similarly charged. Sam and Maisy, my older two children, got in the habit of bringing me coffee while I logged on to our team page every morning. They would hover over my shoulder, then squeal and hug each other to celebrate our most recent tally. Meanwhile, Hadley brought me random coins and pledged daily lemonade stands to support our team. When she learned that wintertime was not good for the lemonade business, she resorted to selling pictures and coloring pages. As for Chris, despite his own full-time career as a beloved pediatrician, he began to take over more and more roles at home to allow me time and freedom to do what I needed to do for the team, the food fight, and the charity. Because he was incapable of sacrificing one bit of the time he devoted to his patients, he began sacrificing his own free time for me. In fact, he seemed to plop his own running on a figurative couch just like the one he had yanked me off of all those years before.

By early February, one month after the team was started, none of the people associated with us even tried to suppress their excitement. Instead, we all made shameless efforts to draw every patient, friend, employee, and acquaintance into our fold.

While Team CMMD did not have a geographic home, we had a virtual one. Our team, made up of people from all walks of life and all parts of the country, gathered on our Facebook page. There, the daily conversations kept us laughing, crying, and, above all, motivated. Besides veteran and would-be runners, we found ourselves collecting a vast number of supporters. All sorts of people who had heard of our team through runners, friends, and friends of runners "liked" our Facebook fan page to keep abreast of our progress. These non-running supporters would ultimately round out our serving team for the food fight and be indispensable contributors to our team effort.

Tom and I took our rivalry to new levels as I found myself scheming about ways to sabotage him, fully expecting that he was doing the same. I tried to pull hints of his plan out of Amy, but she was tight lipped. I was her boss, but for this throwdown, she was firmly on her husband's side. The war between Tom and me had turned ruthless. It was shameful, brutal, and so very exhilarating.

Before long, we learned that our rivalry, slightly contrived as it was, was gaining a lot of attention. People loved watching our interactions on Facebook and in person. Slowly but surely, our collective sea of supporters began to divide, and each of us developed a die-hard following. One of our greatest challenges was to keep the atmosphere between us electrified while keeping our dishes absolutely secret. For this contest to be truly fair, it had to be blind. However, because our guests had paid a lot of money for tickets and would be eating a lot of food in one night, it was very important that our dishes be at least somewhat compatible. The last thing we wanted was to serve five identical courses or, worse, ten completely incompatible dishes. So Tom and I would be forced to share our menus with each other.

We agreed to meet to discuss the final menus at the Blue Cafe. Once we both accepted the courses, the rule was that no significant changes could be made. We sat stone-faced in a booth as Pauly poured us strong coffee from a glass carafe. His own white apron was covered in set-in splotches only partially concealed by fresh, red raspberry coulis stains. Pauly's raspberry coulis could make *any* dish better. He not only would be our gracious host, having agreed to turn his restaurant over for a night, but also would serve as a neutral advisor to us both.

Despite the seeming simplicity of his breakfast-and-lunch café, Pauly also happened to be a renowned sommelier, having worked at some of our area's most lauded restaurants. We decided to add a layer to our already-complex planning: Pauly would choose reasonably priced wines to pair with each course. We hoped that we would be able to use some wines repeatedly with different courses to keep our servers' nearly inconceivable responsibilities as simple as possible. It was going to be hard enough for a group of people who had never so much as laid eyes on one another, much less worked together, to serve these ten plates quickly and efficiently. Adding wine pouring and glass swapping just might break them. Ultimately, Pauly chose five different wines that would be poured according to detailed instructions we would give our servers on the night of the event.

I was so intimidated by Pauly. Like Tom, he was a tall, bearded, and bald man. Compared with their heft and booming voices, I felt tiny. I couldn't stop my hands from shaking as I pulled out my menu that morning at the Blue Cafe, although inwardly I laughed at myself. As a medical student on surgical rotation, I had held a pulsing aorta with more confidence. I took a breath and launched into a detailed description of my menu.

My plan was to start the meal with a single seared shrimp garnished with the same homemade fried tortillas and mango salsa that Tom had tasted and corrected years ago. It was so fitting. He growled a little as I smiled while describing my mango salsa, "emboldened by just a hint of fresh cilantro." Next, my guests would be served a carrot soup flavored with the same Egyptian spices I grew up with: cumin, coriander, and cayenne. I had already made the soup several times but was just not happy with the final result. The color was wrong.

"Um, I have a question about my carrot soup, Pauly," I stammered. "It has this funky brownish color—it's not very vibrant or appealing to the eye. Any ideas what I could do to fix that?"

"You gotta blanch those carrots and plunge 'em in an ice bath—you'll get your orange, all right. And if that's not enough, put a drop of orange food coloring in every batch."

Tom sat up with indignation. "What? You cannot use food coloring!"

"Show me where that rule is," I countered, as I added orange food coloring to my shopping list.

After soups, salads would be served to freshen the palates and prepare folks for the heavier entrées to come. *Gargeer* (pronounced *gar-gear*), Arabic for arugula, was often served alongside heavier dishes to add freshness to meals. In fact, it was a widely held belief in Egyptian households that if you served a bunch of gargeer to guests, they would eat more and leave with fuller bellies—the truest sign of being loved and happy. Some way or another, *gargeer* was going to appear in my salad. I had concocted a lemon vinaigrette over the last year and knew it could dress a bed of arugula. I also had gotten into pickling all sorts of things, from traditional vegetables and fruits to nontraditional things like hard-boiled eggs and turnips. At one point, my son ran from me, pretending to shield his pencil eraser. "No, Mom, I need this eraser. You are not allowed to pickle it!"

As I planned my salad, I remembered one of Tant's favorite meals: *gibna bi batikh* (pronounced *gib-na bi but-teekh*)—cheese with watermelon. Like so many of those lazy summer lunches I remembered having in Cairo, *gibna bi batikh* was beautiful in its simplicity. No matter what feast she had toiled to prepare for us, Tant would often settle for a chunk of salty table cheese, like feta, and a few cubes of chilled watermelon. She would even eat the white rind just beneath the skin. But since it was the dead of winter in Pennsylvania, fresh watermelon would be neither plentiful nor appropriate for our food fight, so I decided to attempt to pickle a watermelon rind and add a bit of warm, crispy goat cheese to the bed of arugula. Fresh pomegranate seeds and crispy pancetta would serve as garnishes.

As I described my salad to Pauly, he frowned. "Now, I don't mean to dissuade you, but you got a whole lotta problems with that salad. First of all, not everybody likes arugula; how about mixing in some spinach? And how in the hell are you going to seed enough pomegranates to plate over one hundred salads?"

I had to tread carefully with Pauly. As generous as he was being with his place and his time, he was also old-school about some things. While I was striving to preserve the integrity of the menu I had created, I had a deep respect for Pauly and his experience, so I promised to take his thoughts under advisement. At that moment, I could not bring myself to explain to Pauly and Tom the reason why I could never, ever put spinach in that salad.

Tant had a spinach phobia. Well, it was more like a superstition. For years, every time she cooked spinach or *sabanikh* (pronounced *sab-an-ick*) in any form, something bad happened. At the massive seventh-birthday party for her son, she served *golash bi sabanikh*—spinach-stuffed phyllo triangles. Just before the cake, my cousin fell and broke his arm. At a family gathering over Christmas, a guest brought a classic spinach pie. Later that night, someone tripped and landed on my aunt's glass coffee table, shattering it in a million pieces. The last time spinach ever appeared on Tant's table—simmered with garlic and tomatoes— her mother ended up hospitalized with the leukemia that years later claimed her life. From that day on, not only did my aunt refuse to cook spinach, but she did not allow it in her house in any shape or form. *No, Pauly. There will be no spinach in my salad.*

The shrimp, soup, and salad would all be opening acts before my headliner: braised beef short ribs garnished with tomato jam and crispy fried shallots. Thanks to Chris, I had gotten the short ribs just right. They would be tender and rich. The tomato jam would cut that richness, while the crispy shallots would add just the right amount of crunch. I imagined the beef nestled into a bed of the creamiest, most decadent whipped potatoes.

Again, Pauly gave me a dubious look. "You ever made home-made mashed potatoes for a hundred people before?" He obviously knew I hadn't.

Tom felt the momentary edge and piped up. "Oh, hey, don't worry, Christine—just add boxed potato flakes to your list—right under the orange food coloring."

We all laughed, and for the moment the situation was diffused. In addition to the impracticality of pomegranate seeds, I would have to think about those potatoes.

The dessert course had me stumped for a while as well. If I had to choose one dessert that defined me, it was cake. In the days before our meeting with Pauly, I contemplated cake as an option for my dessert. It certainly had its advantages: I could easily make a lot of it and could do so ahead of time. The only problem was that I happened to be a terrible baker. In fact, the only cakes I ever made were the boxed variety. I had very strong feelings about cake, not unlike my aunt's adamant stance on spinach. Because Duncan Hines yellow cake with chocolate frosting was so dear to me, I hated the thought of tarnishing its memory with my hopeless baking skills—especially on such an important night. Besides, the idea of trying to pass off boxed cake as home-made to people paying $60 a head for their meal just didn't sit right with me.

* * *

Chris and I had known each other less than three months when my twenty-second birthday rolled around. In preparation for a blind birthday date with another guy, I wriggled into my black jeans, which contrasted nicely with my gold sequined tank top and matching four-inch hoop earrings. Plastic pick and two-thirds of a can of hairspray later, and I had my coif teased to perfection. *Oh, yeah. Hot. Jersey. Med. Student. On. The. Loose.*

My blind date was a disaster. I came home to my tiny studio apartment despondent, hair flat and feet aching from my faux-leather clogs. My answering-machine light was blinking, and I thanked God for that; med school had turned out to be quite lonely and full of cutthroat competition and endless studying.

A message from the cute guy downstairs perked me right up. After a few rides in the elevator, run-ins in the library, and the occasional bite to eat after anatomy, Chris and I had become fast friends. He was just who I needed to hear from on this disappointing birthday.

"Hey . . . uh . . . I . . . know you are out with a guy on a date and stuff like that . . . but I . . . uh . . . well, wanna come down for a bit when you get back? Cool . . . Catchya."

Yes. That was his message, verbatim.

He certainly was not the most eloquent fellow. *"Catchya?" Really? Catch me where? What am I? A fish? And are you so busy after that pathetic message that you can't complete the thought with the word "later"?*

Snap out of my gum and tease out of my hair, I sighed heavily and headed down the six flights to the ninth floor, where Chris's own miniature apartment was. As I reached number 914, I heard the strum of a guitar. The music was coming from inside the apartment. The chords were unmistakable. It was "Blood and Fire," one of my favorite Indigo Girls songs. I think I knew at that moment that I could *really* get to like this guy.

In response to my timid knock, he called out, "Yo!"

Jesus. Why am I here? Just what this hot mama needed—another boring encounter with some random dude, and on her birthday!

I took a deep breath and pushed the door open. The apartment was so cozy and *clean*. It smelled like . . . like . . . cake? Chris got up from the hideous brown striped couch in his living-studying-eating area. It took him a long time to take the guitar pick out of his mouth. I frowned at the godforsaken flannel shirt he was wearing. Later, I would learn that he had dozens of those shirts.

Yet, despite his social ineptitude, in his smiling blue eyes, I found, for the first time, a comfort that, even to this day, can fix anything. As if we were old friends, I found myself kicking off my shoes and flopping down on his couch.

As I regurgitated the disastrous details of my date, my soon-to-be-best friend snuck into his tiny kitchen and emerged with a nicely frosted, layered birthday cake—yellow on the inside, chocolate on the outside—adorned with a single flickering candle. "Ah, it was just a Duncan Hines box," he explained. "I just think everybody should have a cake on their birthday!" I think I knew at *that* moment I would marry this guy.

We talked and laughed for hours about how his mom had bought him cake pans, a mixer, and a frosting spatula. She must have thought that while he was studying to be a doctor, the need for a homemade cake would arise. Chris cringed as I told him about how my date thought a fun thing to do would be to attend a youth meeting and then participate in a covered-dish supper in a church basement. I had just declined the guy's invitation to go bowling when I got the message to meet Chris.

"Huh." He smiled. "If you had gone bowling, that could have actually been the most pathetic birthday story I have ever heard!" We laughed and ate cake, and slowly but surely I fell in love.

*　*　*

Duncan Hines yellow cake with chocolate frosting had become an annual birthday tradition at home. I had such wonderful memories of those twenty-plus cakes Chris and I had shared that I needed to leave that cake off my menu. I had to come up with a dessert that reminded me of my aunt and yet would appeal to the masses. As great as Egyptian food was, we were not known for decadent desserts.

Finally, I got it. I remembered those sultry summers in Cairo as a kid. My aunt would walk me down the busy street to the vendor selling *gelati*, a huge, thick ice cream bar on a stick. She would stop in the middle of the sidewalk and bend down to wipe the creamy, French-style vanilla and melting chocolate shell off my face. Nothing ever tasted better to me than that ice cream bar, except maybe Duncan Hines yellow cake with chocolate frosting.

"I am making ice cream for dessert," I told Pauly and Tom. "Salted caramel with homemade chocolate-covered pretzels."

I did not give Pauly a chance to discourage me. "I know, I know—I have to make a lot of ice cream."

All of a sudden, Pauly was ducking into his kitchen and emerging with two wooden barrels. "I have ice cream makers!" he declared proudly.

Tom and I looked at each other. Even for this tasting menu, I would need to make at least fifty cups of ice cream. We would have to run and refreeze the bowls on those one-quart makers at least a dozen times. It would take me literally two weeks to make all that ice cream, and that option was out of the question.

I left Pauly's feeling like my fabulous menu needed a ton of work. One of my biggest problems with the whole menu was going to be that ice cream. As much as I hated to admit it, I feared I might have to scrap that plan altogether.

Later that night, as I reviewed the team roster, it occurred to me that one of the elite runners on our team owned several Dairy Queen franchises. Not only had she finished Broad Street in the top five of her age category, but Nicole Okolowicz, like most of us, was a cancer hater and wanted to do anything possible to support our team. I e-mailed her to see if I could bring my ice cream base—the thickened custard made by combining eggs, sugar, milk, and cream—to one of her stores the day before the food fight just to freeze it in one of the machines.

"Ugh!" she replied. "I would love to help you, but you can only put Dairy Queen mixes in those machines. Now, if you want to use our vanilla base and mix in some candy or something . . ."

No way. I might have been willing to use food coloring,

but powdered potatoes and premade ice cream base were out of the question.

Fortunately, ice cream professionals, like doctors, are a tight bunch, and Nicole was able to reach out to the owner of our local MaggieMoo's. As soon as Mike McGonagle heard our story, he called me. "Doc, I would love to help! Consider one of my ice cream freezers yours. Just bring me your base, and we can get those thirteen quarts churned in under thirty minutes. But let me ask you an important question: Have you thought about how you are going to store all that ice cream?"

Shit. I hadn't thought of the massive freezer space I would need. Mike laughed. "No worries. I will set aside a freezer just for your ice cream, and how about I throw in some commercial ice cream pans? They will keep the ice cream frozen out of the freezer for up to four hours. That should make serving all those people a breeze."

I explained that because we were trying to raise money for a charity, I really could not afford to pay him.

"Hey, listen, both my parents died of cancer. Cancer just blows. I'll settle for a taste of that salted caramel—it sounds awesome!"

The final piece of the puzzle for me was figuring out whether I had the time and labor available to include mashed potatoes and pomegranate seeds in my five-course meal. As soon as word of our proposed contest was out, my inbox was flooded by people offering hands and help. I decided to call in all those favors. I would enlist a few enthusiastic teammates to seed pomegranates and peel potatoes. Pauly was right that they were tedious and unmanageable tasks for me—but not with help. And, if nothing else, this team knew how to lend a hand.

The weekend after the meeting with Pauly, our menus were set in stone. I issued a call to anyone on the team who might be interested in helping the night of the food fight. I asked any willing and able volunteers to come to a critical strategy meeting the very next weekend at my house, starting at noon sharp. The week flew by as I made shopping lists, prep lists, and timelines. I didn't hear much from the team about intentions to show up for the meeting, and the night before, I was very nervous, as I realized Tom and I might be the only people present.

Tom arrived first, with two trays of hoagies, four bags of chips, and dozens of cans of soda. "Where is everybody?" he asked.

I was about to break the news to him that we had way too much food and no one was coming, when the doorbell rang. The three runners on the porch had not even gotten their coats off when three more appeared. Within a few moments, I realized that I had to just hold the door open. Runner after runner marched in. They hugged me, hugged Tom, then hugged each other. I recognized a few faces, but not most.

By 12:10, every chair and counter space in my kitchen had a person perched on it. People stretched out on the floor and sat Indian-style in my adjoining family room. As I looked around, I counted forty-three people. I could not speak, for fear of breaking down. I looked pleadingly at Tom, hoping he would take my hint and start the meeting. Instead, he said, "Wow. There are a lot of freaking people in here!"

Chapter 7: CATARACTS AND NATURE'S FRIDGE

Patience is bitter, but its fruit is sweet.

—Aristotle

When the alarm went off at 2:45 A.M., I had been in bed for less than an hour. Chris groaned and shifted but showed no other signs of life. I was acutely aware of three things: pounding in my head, throbbing in my knees, and raw, blistering pain in my hands. I lay on my back for a second, trying to summon the energy to get out of bed. The pain in my palms willed me to lift my arms toward my face, but I couldn't see anything.

Chris was snuffling beside me in the pitch darkness. Any tiny glimmer emanating from a clock, DVD player, or even the power button of my laptop could keep him up, so he often woke up in the night and threw random coverings on any such light source. The alarm was still buzzing insistently; I reached over blindly to turn it off. As exhausted as I was, I knew Chris was tired, too. The food fight, the ubiquity of the team, and our Broad Street Run training had really impacted every aspect of our lives together. I expected to be tired, but he deserved at least one full night's sleep.

The alarm button was obscured by some bit of fabric. I wasn't surprised to see that, but I was surprised to find that on this particular night Chris had chosen a bikini top out of my swimsuit drawer to cover the clock. Pushing the *he's nuts* thoughts out of my mind were wistful memories of the last time I had worn that bikini, nearly nine months earlier. At that moment, in the wee hours of the morning on February 23, 2013, nothing seemed farther away than the turquoise waters of Turks and Caicos, the exclusive Caribbean islands we had visited just before I learned of Tant's sickness, and the home of the most beautiful beaches I had ever seen.

Impatiently, I threw the bathing suit on the floor and swung my legs over the side of the bed. I was still in my jeans and long-sleeved Tshirt. The filthy apron I seemed never to be without restricted my movement just enough to remind me that I hadn't bothered to take it off before collapsing on the bed.

It wasn't until I was in the bathroom that I finally saw my hands. Both palms were swollen and red. The skin on the pads of my fingers was peeling. The burn marks from the oven grates created a pattern on my hands as complex as a topographic map of Everest. The cool water splashing on my face did little to wake me, but it did cool the pain in my hands—at least for the moment.

I trudged down the steps to the same kitchen that I seemed

just to have left. Full of braising short ribs, both ovens were humming. The lights were dim, and I intentionally did not brighten the room. My head was still throbbing and seemed to be keeping time with the pounding in my heart. Exhaustion was not enough to temper the nervousness that had consumed me over the last few days.

As I lifted the foil from the corner of one of the pans, I was rewarded with a cloud of unctuous steam that immediately gave away the ingredients of my braising liquid: garlic, ginger, tomatoes, and soy sauce. When I pierced the nearest piece of meat with my testing fork, it met with the slightest resistance.

I sighed. They were not ready yet. Maybe another hour.

I reached for the nearest dish towel and began what had become my "rotating" ritual. In order to ensure even cooking, I moved the pans from top to bottom oven shelf and from left to right. I had long given up on any systematic approach and just shuffled the pans around, hoping every one ended up in a different spot. The night before, two of my three sous chefs, Arlen and James, had meticulously lined the seared short ribs into roasting pan after roasting pan. The spacing was critical. Crowding the meat together would not allow for proper circulation of the liquid and some pieces would end up dry. Placing the short ribs too far apart would distort the delicate meat: liquid ratio and the short ribs would end up boiling instead of braising.

Once I had approved each pan, we had poured the cooking liquid over the top. Just before we'd covered the pans and slid them into the hot ovens, I had done some mental math.

In the weeks before the food fight, when I had tested the short-rib recipe for the five of us at home, the meat had become fork tender in about three hours. Now, I figured the sheer volume of food and liquid would necessitate a slightly longer cooking time—maybe four and a half hours—so I had filled the ovens at 7:00, thinking they would need until midnight, at the latest, to be done properly.

By midnight, I had been dying to get into bed. The last forty-eight hours had been full of nonstop prep work for what could be the most important meal of my life. But, despite my careful calculations, the ribs had been nowhere near ready, so I'd decided to leave them in and check on them every forty-five minutes or so, trying to steal bits of sleep between inspections. This 2:45 A.M. check was the third time I had hauled myself out of bed to find that the ribs were still not ready.

I felt tears stinging my eyes as I slammed the oven door shut. I resisted the temptation to pull them out and just be done. No one would notice. What did it matter? It was a ridiculous contest—the whole thing was going to be a huge flop. As I fought the negativity, I thought of my aunt and her meticulousness in the kitchen, in her work, and in her life. She took the same measured approach with her twentieth patient of the day as she did with her first. It was a lesson I learned from her early on. "If you cram thirty people into my schedule," I had recently explained to my staff, "not only is it not fair to me, it's not fair to the patient—I am not good for patient number thirty, who deserves as much of me as patient number one."

Tant, on the other hand, never complained—and she didn't need to give her staff complicated scheduling rules. She just did what she had to do and gave every last patient what they needed.

She would have given me a knowing look if she had seen

me pull that meat out a minute too soon. I could hear her voice: *Cat, not yet. All this time, and you're going to ruin them over one more hour?*

Suddenly, I missed her desperately and reached for my phone, only to be halted by the glaring time on its screen: 3:00 A.M. A call from me at this hour would scare her to death. Besides, she needed all the rest she could get right now. I wondered if she had ever almost given up on her treatments. She had just finished her last chemo a few days before. After six months, I was sure, she was weary. But, knowing her, I was sure she'd stuck it out even in the last hours. If she could do that, I could certainly cook some short ribs overnight.

Once I had basted the meat, sealed the foil, and rotated the pans, I flopped down at the kitchen table. Despite the starless winter darkness, I could make out the drifts of snow on our deck. I had never been so glad about a cold snap as I had been about our most recent one, which had brought nearly six inches of snow and consistently low temperatures. Across the deck, orange five- and ten-gallon buckets were nestled in the deep white snow. Giant black letters scrawled hastily on the sides and lids identified the contents: "tomato jam—ready, just reheat"; "potatoes—peeled, in salt water, need cubing"; "carrot soup—pureed, needs cream, test seasoning."

In the excitement over the instantaneous sellout of our food fight tickets, my feverish menu planning, and my frantic recipe testing, I had neglected to consider one very important thing: refrigerator space. Even if I commandeered every inch of space in all three of our fridges, as well as our neighbors', it would never be enough for the veritable mountains of food we had to prep.

The idea to use "nature's fridge" to store our perishables in the days before the food fight could be credited to one person: my father. It had been scarcely two weeks since his "quick" visit had turned into an extended stay. The evening he had been due to arrive, I had tried to quell the uneasiness in my stomach as dusk turned to night and I realized that the wet roads were probably icing over. My father should have shown up over an hour earlier.

Just as I was about to ask Chris to go out looking for him, the phone rang. "Cat, it's Dad. I am lost, *habibti*."

My heart leaped at the sound of his voice. No matter what, he wasn't dead or, worse, standing me up.

The same feeling of dread that seemed to be lodged in my belly that night had also hit me nearly thirty years before. I was in eighth grade and had been chosen to give a speech, about a class trip to New York City, at a school program one evening. As I took my place at the podium, I scanned the full auditorium for any sight of my father. My disappointment did not hinder my performance, and I concluded the flawless five-minute presentation to loud applause. About an hour later, my mother and I got home to find my dad in his usual chair, the brown faux-suede upholstery worn thin after decades of his weary head resting on it.

"Where were you?" I croaked.

He looked wounded. "What? I was there! I was just late!"

I rolled my eyes as my mother squeezed my shoulder in an attempt to silence what were sure to be volatile words.

"No. No. I really was there," he pleaded.

As I ran up the steps, hot tears streaming down my face, I heard him say quietly, "I got there just in time to hear some girl talking about New York City."

As she wiped the tears off my cheeks, my mother explained, "It's his eyes, *habibti*. He really does not see very well."

Thirty years before, my father's notoriously bad vision had caused me a disappointment I would never forget. That same hopelessly bad vision would ultimately save our food fight.

"Where are you?" I asked when he called, barely hiding the relief in my voice.

After a minute or two, we were able to identify that my father was at Wawa, a common convenience store in Pennsylvania. This one was less than a mile away from our house. He still did not have a cell phone and had been driving around, looking for a pay phone. He didn't want us to go get him.

"Just sit tight," he said. "I should be there in a minute."

Two hours later, he pulled into the driveway just as I was about to dial the police. Chris had already been in and around every convenience store in a five-mile radius, with no luck. Before he was out of the car, we riddled my father with questions. Had we gotten it wrong? Had he been at a different Wawa—one in the next state, perhaps? Like my mother's firm grip on my shoulder all those years before, the look of terror on his face silenced the smart comments on the tip of my tongue. He was late because he couldn't see.

As the sun had set and the glare from the wet roads and headlights had merged, he'd been barely able to see just ahead of him—much less to read street signs. And I was fairly certain the old van he was driving didn't come standard with GPS.

The next morning, I made a call to my ophthalmologist. "Of course I'll see your dad today," he insisted. A few hours later, Dad was diagnosed with bilateral, severe cataracts. He was essentially blind. The surgery could not wait and was scheduled for the following week. Since I trusted my doctor implicitly and since Dad would not be able to drive for a few weeks, we all agreed that he would stay with us until both eyes were done.

His first surgery took place two weeks before the food fight, and the second eye just a week later. So, largely by coincidence, my father ended up being present for the entire food fight planning and preparation process. For the most part, he sat by quietly, but occasionally I caught him smiling a little or chuckling at the repartee between Tom and me, such as on one afternoon when Tom was talking about the goat cheese pudding he planned for dessert. "It will have a rhubarb puree on the bottom and fresh berries on top," he said excitedly.

I stopped dead in my tracks and, forgetting that my father was sitting a few feet away, blurted out, "Where the hell are you going to get rhubarb in February, you dumbass?"

Tom's loud chortle reminded me that my father was there, just in time for me to hear Dad say quietly, "Frozen. You can only find frozen rhubarb this time of year."

Tom, clutching his pen and pad, went over to the couch where my father sat. He leaned in, as if getting the secret of the grail. I shook my head. "Whose side are you on anyway, Dad?" I called happily.

The next day, he overheard my team discussing the mathematics of making enough of five different dishes—some with half a dozen components—to feed over one hundred guests, plus some allowance for error. It was then that he really spoke up.

"*Beebel!*" he began.

I cringed as three patients-teammates turned toward his

broken English. Despite having been in the United States for nearly forty-five years, he still confused *p* and *b* sounds.

"Good job with the math, but . . . Well, I'm just an old man, but . . . Where are you going to put all this food?"

This time the silence wasn't awkward; it was the result of our utter speechlessness. We had no idea how to answer his question.

James went first. "What about the ice cream guy—didn't he say he had a freezer for you?"

"Yes, but he's already holding the ice cream. Besides, we don't need any more freezer room; we need refrigerator space."

Just then, Chris sauntered into the kitchen. In general, he had avoided most of the recent gatherings and meetings. I could see that he was growing tired of the constant intrusions on our home and family—not to mention my utter absence as a mom over the last weeks. Besides that, he had always been shy around my dad.

Chris must have been reading my mind as I mentally cleared our household fridges of their contents. He caught my eye and said firmly, "No, Cat. We actually continue to live in this house, despite the run and the food fight and the team. You cannot empty all of our refrigerators. Your children have school and lunches and will need to eat the occasional meal that does not come out of a box or a paper bag."

Despite his solid logic and his everpresent smile, his words stung. But, as with my sore knee, my piling charts, and countless other things that threatened to derail me from my path to May 5, I brushed off his words. I looked to the others on my team for ideas.

"Pauly?" asked Loretta. The few words she uttered were always soft and carefully chosen; I got the feeling she was sort of nervous around me.

"No," I said, a little too harshly. I threw her a meek, apologetic look and went on. "Pauly was very clear. *His* life and business go on, too." I couldn't help but remember Chris's words from a few minutes before.

"We have access to the restaurant only from 3:00 the afternoon of the food fight until 4:00 early the next morning, when his Sunday breakfast prep begins, and we need to be out of his place without a trace—as in spotless."

My father had wandered in from the family room and stood with his hands behind his back, surveying the view from our back deck. It was always gorgeous in the winter. From our perch on top of a hill, the lights of the town below sparkled like holiday decorations. It wouldn't be until the trees filled in around April that we would lose that vista. My heart skipped, and instantly I identified the feeling in my chest. It was pride. As my father stood quietly, I sent a silent message to him. *Yes, Dad. I live here in this beautiful house on top of this big hill. I have patients and friends who love me enough to be here at midnight, sorting this stuff out. And you know what's nuts? I'm really glad you're here with us.*

His soft tapping on the glass broke my reverie, and the words I wanted to say were trampled by the ones he uttered aloud: "It's right here—your refrigerator."

I looked out at the deck, fully outfitted with a grill, chaise lounges, a huge table, and an umbrella. Below, the circular patio had been cleared of its furnishings, except for the fire pit.

There was no fridge.

Suddenly, James pushed his chair back and jumped up. "Yes! Of course! We will put everything outside. As long as there isn't risk of freezing, and as long as we're really careful to protect everything from raccoons and deer, that should be fine."

We glanced at the forecast and saw that temperatures were expected to hold steady in the mid-thirties for the rest of the week. We were giddy. Thanks to my dad, we had just found 1,500 square feet of empty fridge space—literally outside the kitchen door. I remembered that I had used five-gallon buckets from Home Depot to brine turkeys in years past. They were easy to find, and inexpensive—the logical vessel for the huge volumes of food we would be preparing.

* * *

These were the very buckets that dotted the snow-covered deck that early morning before the food fight. The sight of them lifted my spirits, and I suddenly had the second wind I needed. At 3:30 A.M., I made coffee and pulled out my laptop. It was time to run the food offerings one by one until I could recite the prep lists, plating notes, and dish descriptions.

I thought back to how far my menu had come since that first meeting with Pauly, six weeks before. I had stood my ground— no powdered potatoes would come within a mile of my meal. It was amazing how this challenge and those five dishes had since taken on a life of their own—molded not just by me, but by my three sous chefs.

I recalled the tasting meeting I had called for my kitchen team. I had created every component of each of my five dishes. I had visualized each plate and had a picture of it in my mind. I had tested, tasted, reworked, and retasted the recipes until their flavor, texture, portion, and presentation were all up to my standards.

Or so I thought.

With a great deal of slightly exaggerated humility, I gathered my three assistants around my island.

"Appetizer," I announced. "I am calling this a shrimp *taquito*. A lime-marinated, seared shrimp will be placed atop a lightly griddled miniature tortilla. The shrimp will be topped with a fresh mango salsa, and the plate will be dressed with crisscrossing ribbons of avocado cream and sriracha crème fraîche. Lastly, two thin, handfried tortilla strips will be placed on top."

With a flourish, I placed the completed plate in the middle of the otherwise-empty island. I had always loved this dish. I waited for the oohs and aahs.

None came.

As if they'd rehearsed, James, Arlen, and Loretta leaned forward in synchrony. James reached over and fondled the shrimp, Arlen scraped my salsa off to the side, and Loretta boldly swiped a finger through the sauces. As she pondered the flavors with her eyes shut, Arlen and James fired comments at me: "Shrimp is overcooked." "Salsa is watery and not spicy enough." "Tortilla is dry."

I looked to Loretta for her usual gentle words. None came. "Um. I think that the sauces are not flavorful enough. They don't really pop on your tongue. They need to tie the whole thing together—not sure they do that." She pushed the dissected plate toward her compatriots.

As I stared at what was left of my creation, I thought of

how my cadavers had looked after a session of gross anatomy in medical school. How could something so spectacular as the human body be reduced to shreds of unidentifiable sinews and scraps? Apparently, it was a lot like my shrimp plate.

James did not mince words. "I got the creams. I can stop wars with my sauces. Gimme two days, and I'll bring you a sample that will bring Tom to his knees."

Once the shock of their preliminary, loveless reactions passed, I felt relieved. Even though I had never cooked with James, I was inexplicably confident that he would absolutely rock those sauces.

The news did not get better as my courses advanced. The carrot soup was "grainy and gray," although the idea of serving it in an espresso cup was "great." The arugula was not crisp enough, and the goat cheese needed to be warm, not cold. They agreed that the dressing was light and delicious but that it would need a very delicate hand to apply it. As we contemplated which of us would take on this critical salad task, they announced unanimously, "Anyone but Christine." Apparently, I had not adhered to my own "less is more" dressing mantra. "Hey! Is that watermelon rind? Pickled?" James asked. "Genius!"

I barely hid my pout as my hands moved on to the main course. My score with the pickle was not quite enough to heal all the other hurts. As I assembled my entrée plate, they watched over my shoulder. And, as I now expected, questions flew: "Are you serving in a bowl? Good—catch all the sauce." "Are those potatoes going to be prewhipped? Bad idea. They need to be made last-minute."

The sight of the succulent strips of beef being pulled from

the bubbling braising liquid finally stopped the chatter. I topped off my plate with the slow-cooked tomato jam—it really should have been called painfully slow-cooked, as it had taken more than nine hours to turn mountains of fresh tomatoes into the thick, slightly sweet, slightly sour jam with just the right level of tang and richness.

Next, I dropped a handful of battered shallot rings into oil that had been quietly coming to temperature. After a minute, I pulled them out of the oil, dabbed them on a paper towel, and hit them with a few grains of sea salt. Carefully, I placed them on top of the small mound of jam. Finally, I poured the sauce: a clarified, reduced, thinner version of the braising liquid. It had all the same flavors as the liquid that the beef had cooked in but was lighter and cleaner, after having been strained three times to remove impurities. This sauce was meant to just moisten the fluffy mound of potatoes and bring all the flavors of the dish together.

As the sauce dripped from my ladle into the small bowl, all three groaned. "No. No! Why would you do that?" "The potatoes will run!" "There's too much sauce and it is too thin!" "What if it sloshes around when the inexperienced servers slap the bowls down on the tables?"

My exhaustion and disappointment nearly got the better of me. I was about to throw my hands up and send them all home, when I noticed that suddenly the room was quiet. I looked up to see my assistants each with a mouthful of beef and potato and sauce. They crunched the shallots and savored the tomato jam.

Finally, someone—I don't remember who—spoke. "Holy shit. This kicks ass. This plate—this is your ticket, right here."

I was so relieved that the things we needed to do to the entrée were essentially cosmetic that I distractedly pulled out a handful of spoons and a quart of my salted caramel ice cream. I didn't have time to scoop it and garnish it. The three were digging in before the freezer door was even shut. Once again, for an agonizing minute, no one spoke.

This time, it was Arlen. "The greatest master chefs are brought down on desserts. You, my friend, have just won this contest—on dessert."

* * *

That morning before we were due to serve our meals, I remembered that initial tasting and all the work we had done on those five dishes in the weeks since. Suddenly, warm self-assurance washed over me. This menu had gone from good to better to nearly flawless. The flavors were right, and the plating was impeccable. It was finally game time. It was time to win this thing for my aunt.

At 4:30 on the morning of the food fight, I finally shut down my laptop. Our last-minute preparations for the highly anticipated contest would begin in two hours. I needed to shut my eyes for just a few minutes. . . .

Chapter 8: MISSING CILANTRO

Perseverance is not a long race; it is

many short races one after the other.

—Walter Elliott

The quiet clanging of metal and glass woke me. Arlen had come in through the front door. Anticipating that my team would arrive early, I had left it unlocked. I opened my eyes and looked up at the ceiling. I didn't remember lying down, but it was apparent that sometime after 4:30 A.M., I had fallen asleep on the family-room couch. My neck was stiff, and I tried awkwardly to look at the enormous mantel clock without turning my head. It was exactly 6:00 A.M. Our first guests were due to arrive at the Blue Cafe in thirteen hours.

It had become clear a few weeks before that I would need to delegate some of the tasks associated with this event. I had sent a mass e-mail asking for volunteers and had been flooded with responses. Elaine, a bubbly, fun-loving woman who had lost her mother to ovarian cancer, offered to coordinate all the volunteers. We had three volunteer bartenders. Their job was simply to pour wine, as that was the only alcohol we planned on serving. We even secured three dishwashers. Amy, Tom's wife, and Karen Baker, the sarcoma survivor who had been booted out of a local restaurant while on her quest for donations, took charge of the silent auction. A dozen people, most of them patients, volunteered to wait tables. Leigh and her design team set to work on the menus and ballots.

It was partly because of these volunteers that, as I lay there on the couch after my nap, I felt lighter and clearer. Those ninety minutes of sleep had done wonders for my state of mind. The angst and negativity of the night before were gone and had left an eerie confidence in their place. It no longer occurred to me that a volunteer might not show up or that something would be forgotten.

It wasn't until I was upright and I heard Arlen call, "Good morning, sunshine!" that the magnitude of our to-do list began to sink in again. I smiled, tucked my feet into my slippers, and jumped up. As I made a halfhearted attempt to smooth my mass of frizzy hair, I marveled at how close we all had become. Arlen started as a patient of mine who had been to the office only a handful of times. As a veteran runner and a closet foodie, he was a natural addition to my running and cooking team. I never would have imagined that one Saturday *any* patient would be standing in my kitchen at 6:00 A.M. while I slept on the couch, yet, on that particular morning, that scenario seemed as natural as could be. He handed me a spoonful of the sauce we would serve with our short ribs. It was perfect.

The counters were covered in containers of all different

shapes and sizes. Everything was sealed with masking tape and labeled with Sharpies. I pulled the massive dry-erase board out of the laundry room and felt my heart pound. Every inch of the five-by-three-foot surface was covered in writing. The tasks were organized according to the times they would need to be started in order for us to stay on schedule. Some things had to be done just minutes before serving, and others could be completed hours before our guests arrived.

As I read through the prep list, I mentally ran through all the courses again. The shrimp *taquito* with fresh salsa would be served first. That salsa could not be made more than a few hours ahead, and all the components had to be chopped by hand. Every ingredient for the salsa was grouped together in the cardboard box I began to inventory: mangoes, tomatoes, red onions, peppers, seasonings, jalapeños, garlic, and half a gallon of freshly squeezed lime juice—the product of the lime-squeezing "party" to which I had invited people two days before, where we had used an electric juicer to extract the liquid from at least a hundred limes.

The produce in the box looked good, but something wasn't right. Something was missing. *Mangoes, peppers, tomatoes . . . What is it?* I called Arlen over. "What's missing from this box?" I asked..

It took him only a moment to answer, "Cilantro. Where's the cilantro? I know I saw it in here the other day. . . ."

The very ingredient Tom had encouraged me to add to my salsa on the night we'd first met, five years before, was not in the box. Cilantro was an indispensable herb, one with such a unique flavor that no substitute existed. Arlen was already putting his coat on. "No worries," he said with authority. "I will be right back with cilantro."

Twenty minutes later, I had gotten through most of the checklist when my cell phone rang. Arlen was calling from the produce section of our local high-end grocery. Wegmans was not just a grocery store; it was a cook's paradise—stocked full of every imaginable fruit, vegetable, and herb in mind-boggling quantities.

"Are you sitting?" Arlen sounded panicked. I blinked and felt my mouth suddenly go dry. "Wegmans is out of cilantro."

How the hell is Wegmans out of anything? I digested the information and began to mentally calculate the amount of precious time we would lose crisscrossing town to find this critical ingredient. Arlen was still talking.

"C, there's this one other thing. Uh . . . now you really ought to be sitting. The produce manager told me that there was some sort of run on cilantro yesterday. Apparently, a tall, bald guy with a beard came in and bought literally every bunch of it off the shelf. They won't be getting more till tomorrow."

Tom. Tom O'Grady bought up every bunch of cilantro in the store. The thought sprang into my mind instantly. I shook my head at the utter craziness of it. *Could he? Would he?*

Days before, my garage had been transformed into a "warehouse" for all of the ingredients and equipment we would need for the contest. Because of that, Tom had been in and out of my house for days. In fact, despite the fact that he was my archnemesis, I had given him the code to the garage opener. He needed to be able to come and go freely. Apparently, that was precisely what he had done. Not only had he lifted the critical ingredient out of my salsa prep box, he had made sure that replacing it would cost my team precious time.

Since Arlen was now out of commission, hunting for my

missing ingredient, I called the rest of my team. "I know it's early, guys, but I need you here *now*."

I then sent a text to my competitor. "It's going to take a lot more than a missing herb to bring me down, mister. But you wanna play dirty? Game on."

My heart quickened as much with excitement over the possibilities of ruining *him* as with fear of what he might have in store for *me*. Part of this competition was going to involve the ability to bounce back and improvise in the face of the unexpected. I was glad for my nap and my coffee. Clearly, I would need both for the physical and mental games we were about to play.

James was the first to arrive. "Two hundred and thirty-five!" he announced triumphantly. The massive bucket full of shrimp he had spent hours cleaning, deveining, and counting hit the floor with a dramatic *clunk*.

"You counted them?" I was unsuccessful at masking the surprise in my voice. As senseless as it seemed at first, James's shrimp counting might have afforded us a weapon capable of undoing the damage the cilantro incident had caused. Originally, we planned on serving one shrimp to each of our 104 guests. Thanks to James, we discovered that, even allowing for a dropped plate or two, we would have enough shrimp to serve *two* to each person.

The day before, as I'd packed spices from my pantry into a shoebox, I had seen a huge bag of shredded coconut. Now it hit me: "Guys! I have an idea!"

All six helpers in my kitchen let out a groan. Arlen had returned with cilantro—it had taken him nearly an hour to find it, but he had it. He spoke gently, verbalizing what everyone in the room was thinking. "C, we really need to focus on what we already have to get done—it's a lot, and we just have to buckle down. . . ." He trailed off, realizing that I was not taking no for an answer.

I practically had to will my feet to stay planted on the floor as my excitement mounted. "Let's do shrimp two ways! We'll make a coated and fried coconut shrimp to go alongside the seared, lime-marinated one. It will be beautiful with the tropical flavors of the salsa, and talk about difficulty—the judges and guests won't miss that."

Loretta was already trying to work out the proportions of coconut to flour for the recipe as I pulled out a huge pot and started filling it with peanut oil, which we'd decided to use for all the frying, as it had a subtle flavor and could tolerate high temperatures without smoking. Now, we needed to experiment. Once we had the coconut shrimp recipe and fry time down, we would prep them, then do the frying at the last minute.

I understood why my team was so reluctant. We were already planning to fry tortilla strips and shallots. Pauly's kitchen did not have a professional-grade deep-fryer, so we would have to use his single, gigantic stockpot filled with oil for all of our frying. If we didn't get the temperature of that oil just right, those little garnishes could ruin the very plates they were meant to enhance. Further, since the shrimp was going to be the first course, the shallots for the entrée would need to be fried *after* the shrimp, and shrimp-flavored oil would result in shrimp-flavored shallots.

The second audible groan from my kitchen team came when I reminded them that as soon as the first course was served, we would need to dump that oil out and get a fresh batch on. It could take an hour to heat up that much oil. In short, adding one more deep-fried component to our already-complex menu seemed like sheer lunacy. But I just knew this coconut-crusted shrimp, with its unexpected crunch and sweetness, would elevate my dish exponentially—we *had* to do it.

I dropped two golden shrimp onto a paper towel. As everyone gathered around, I cut one of the two into bite-size pieces. The second one would be our "plating" shrimp. Once we had the flavor right, we needed to work that second shrimp onto our plate. The crispy coating crunched under my knife, revealing the glistening interior of a nicely cooked shrimp. While I didn't feel the need to taste it—cooking was a craft of all senses, and at that moment, sight and hearing were the only two I needed—I did. The flavor of the coconut shrimp did not disappoint.

Reworking our first course was about as easy as about-facing a luxury liner. Duties were reassigned and prep lists revised. By then, it was nearly 10:00. Chris had just herded the kids out of the house. He would take them to breakfast and then come back to help. He smiled at me as he surveyed the dishes, counters, and sink. He was not just glad that the food fight would be over in a few hours; he was happy to be leaving the disaster that had once been our home kitchen.

Loretta volunteered to break away from the forty shallots she was charged with peeling in order to butterfly and batter 115 shrimp. Realizing our manpower was woefully inadequate, I put a plea out on Facebook. "Extra food fighter hands needed on Team Meyer—please save us!"

Twenty minutes later, Wendy Ford was at my door. She had seen the post and headed right over. Wendy was one of the runners who got nearly as much out of the team as she put in. When she first signed on to run with us, her mother had already survived seven different bouts with cancer. Wendy had never run more than two miles, but, like I had, she had been caught in a downward emotional spiral. Upon seeing one of our team posters in my office, she had been moved to sign up. The next morning, Wendy woke up full of buyer's remorse, but she would not be deterred. Instead, she dove full-on into a novice training plan, doing weekday runs at the school gym where she worked and weekend runs on a dying treadmill in her basement. Even when, in the dead of winter and months before race day, that treadmill died, Wendy was not fazed. She promptly accepted my offer to use our home gym on the weekends.

Seeing Wendy blow into the side door of our house every Sunday afternoon was just as natural as seeing Arlen in my kitchen that Saturday at 6:00 A.M. They, like so many others on the team, were no longer just patients to me—they had become my friends. And, as only a true friend would, Wendy came to my rescue the minute I called for help.

By 2:30, we were ready to move out. Buckets of beef, potatoes, and carrot soup were carefully stacked into the back of my Volvo. Sacks of flour and spices filled every available nook. The last thing I slid into the trunk was the dry-erase board. Just before I slammed the hatch shut, my eye caught the bottom-left-hand corner of the board where the word "dessert" had been scrawled like an afterthought.

Shit, the ice cream!

The weekend before, I had spent two full days preparing my secret weapon. If the contest were close, that ice cream would seal my win, so it needed to be flawless. That meant it had to start with a perfect base, or cooked custard. Making that particular custard was a painstaking process, and I had only ever doubled the recipe. For this dinner, I needed to make several batches. That one complex recipe had required my full attention, as well as every pot in my kitchen. After weeks of testing recipes, I had grown weary of doing mental math, so I'd decided that in order to make the massive quantities I needed without sacrificing quality, I would make the ice cream base the same way I always had: two quarts at a time—washing my favorite pots, strainers, and wooden spoons between each batch.

I began the project by making caramel, simply heating sugar in a dry skillet until it melted and turned a rich amber color. Caramel has to be watched constantly. A second too long, and it will burn. Once the caramel reached the desired color, I added cream. Then I mixed the sputtering, bubbling mass of caramel sauce into a simple egg-, cream-, and milk-based custard that I had cooked separately. That custard was high maintenance in its own right: it had to be stirred continuously, or it would turn into a mass of scrambled eggs. At one point on the day I had set out to make all dozens of batches of ice cream, I grabbed a metal pot handle that had been slowly getting red hot atop an adjacent burner. Moments after I threw the pan and its burned caramel into the sink, Chris came bounding up the steps. I stood at the sink, running cold water over my blistering palm.

"What happened?" Chris's normally sunny expression was clouded. Hadley had been floating around the kitchen all morning. Without looking up from the picture she was busily coloring, she explained to her father, "I'm not sure, Daddy. All I know is, it must've been bad, 'cause Mama said the *s*-word, the *d*-word, *and* the *f*-word."

All told, in one day, I burned my palm and three batches of caramel, scrambled a dozen eggs, and washed the same two pots nine times before I finally had six gallons of ice cream base.

Ten hours after starting, and bleary-eyed from exhaustion, I sealed the ice cream base into two five-gallon buckets and nestled them into the snow on the deck to chill completely overnight. The next morning, I transported the base to MaggieMoo's, the local ice cream shop that had offered to bulk-churn my ice cream. Minutes after it was poured into that ice cream maker, my hard-earned liquid base was transformed. I held my breath, half-expecting some catastrophic failure. But, thankfully, a salted caramel ice cream emerged—lovely in color, texture, and flavor. As he promised, Mike McGonagle, the owner of the store, filled plastic tub after plastic tub with the newly spun ice cream. He then labeled every container with four big black letters: CMMD. He piled them into his empty freezer and gave me a hug. "Don't worry! I'll guard it with my life!"

I knew I would not have time the day of the event to pick it up, so I called on someone who had offered to help. The problem was, now, as I stood outside my car just hours before our cook-off was to start, precious minutes ticking by, I could not remember who had been assigned the all-too-critical duty of ice cream pickup. I pressed my fingers into my forehead, as if I could channel the missing information into my blank mind, but it was no use.

Arlen offered to stop by MaggieMoo's to see if the ice cream was still there. If it were, he would bring it to the café. Just as we were pulling into the parking lot, he called. My heart pounded as I picked up my cell. *What if Tom pulled something with the ice cream? I have no other dessert options, and I spent so much time on it. . . . He wouldn't . . . would he?*

"Good news," Arlen was saying. "Your ice cream was picked up two hours ago, according to Mike here, by a short Indian lady?"

Of course! Weeks before, I had asked Jessy John, one of Chris's partners in his pediatric practice and a dear friend, to be in charge of the ice cream. Precisely as I had instructed her to do, she had picked up all six gallons of semisolid gold and dropped them off at the Blue Cafe. Knowing that the ice cream, and therefore one-fifth of my menu, was secure, freed my mind to concentrate on the long list of tasks required to complete the other four menu items.

After unpacking several carloads' worth of supplies and food in various stages of readiness, we all got to work. The kitchen of the café was tiny, and, despite near-freezing temperatures outside, it was blazing hot. Tom and I quickly chose workstations. His usually hulking frame seemed to have shrunk under the slightest droop in his shoulders. He absently wiped tiny beads of sweat from his forehead with the towel tucked into his apron for that specific purpose.

We both then met with our respective teams to discuss our plan of attack in the four hours before our guests were due. My team was on autopilot. They all knew exactly what they needed to do and when they needed to do it. I floated around, making sure that everything tasted good and was being prepared according to my exact instructions. As I came to the salad-prep area, I checked the dressing, pickles, and pancetta. The goat cheese rounds had been coated in bread crumbs the day before and needed to be seared on the flattop—the gigantic, flat griddle that we had preheated and oiled—just before serving. I grabbed a handful of pomegranate seeds and shoved them in my mouth, then immediately spit them into a napkin.

They were disgusting.

Someone had seeded four big pomegranates but had indiscriminately put all the seeds into the prep bowl. As I ran my fingers through them, I noticed that some of the seeds were not the ruby-red color they were supposed to be and were instead gray and mushy. One bad seed could ruin a salad plate, cost me points, or, worse, make someone sick. My choices were few, but I was determined not to compromise my menu. My salad had been billed as having pomegranate seeds, so it would have pomegranate seeds.

I commandeered a young volunteer whom I did not recognize and asked her to pick through the hundreds of seeds one by one, tossing the bad and keeping the good. The tedious task took her almost an hour. We had lost half of our seeds but still had enough to garnish all the salads if we were very careful. "Three pomegranate seeds per plate, guys—no more than *three*," I announced to my team, as if calling for an emergency evacuation. Everyone looked at me with the sympathetic look one might give a homeless person but wordlessly went about their work.

Half an hour before our guests were due to arrive, I stepped out of the kitchen to address our team of volunteers. My eyes burned from the kitchen heat and exhaustion. I rubbed them and blinked once, then again, not believing what I was seeing. The dining room itself seemed to be twinkling.

The modest breakfast-and-lunch café had been transformed with starched linens, sparkling glasses, and the glimmer of freshly lit votive candles. The auction table was covered with row after row of valuable items. A greeting table had been set up near the front door, and two people were poring over a guest list, making sure that only guests who had purchased tickets would be allowed to enter. Dozens of volunteers, some recognizable, many not, were busy with last-minute preparations. They were all in matching black T-shirts emblazoned with the bright orange food fight logo.

As I stepped into the middle of the room, everyone stopped what they were doing. A split second of silence was broken by the sound of one pair of clapping hands, then another, then a roomful. We hadn't even served the meal, and yet a crowd of friends and strangers stood applauding me.

Just then, a blast of cold air forced me to turn toward the door. Chris was balancing the dozen pizzas we had ordered for the staff dinner. He, too, was wearing a signature food fight shirt. He was there in the shirt, he was there in the room—he was just *there*. Standing in the middle of the applauding crowd, eyes locked with the one who mattered most to me, I was overcome with exhaustion, relief, and love. I buried my face in my hands as my tears began to flow.

Suddenly, I felt an arm around my shoulders, holding me up and holding me close. It was so comforting, but I knew it wasn't Chris. Tom, my competitor, was standing next to me. He, too, had tears in his eyes as he drew me to him. "For my aunt Kathy and your *Tant*, let's do this thing! Oh, and by the way, I hope you're ready—I'm about to *really* give you something to cry about."

Chapter 9: Pig Nipples

Winning isn't everything, but wanting to win is.

—Vince Lombardi

Nothing could have been more at odds with the serenity of the candlelit dining room than the frenzied activity of the kitchen on the night of the food fight. As our volunteers' applause died down, Tom draped his arm around my shoulder in one last gesture of friendship. Then, in a split second, he was shoving me and anyone in his path to the side as his big frame barreled into the kitchen. I had to blink against the unnatural white of overhead lights reflecting off dozens of stainless surfaces. Countless people swarmed around the tiny kitchen, which seemed to be in perpetual motion. While everyone moved quickly and with purpose, their faces held a perpetually stunned look.

To keep the contest fair and our guests blind, we flipped a coin to see who would serve first. The rest of the menu order had been randomly assigned weeks before and was posted all over the kitchen for volunteers, servers, and us to refer to. TJ, our emcee, was a tall, attractive man with a firm handshake and an easy smile. His wife had watched her father die of leukemia and was passionate about helping our team and our cause. In fact she thought nothing of assigning TJ emcee duties, despite a planned business trip that had him arriving, jet-lagged, from Europe just hours before our event. On the flight home, TJ had carefully rehearsed elaborate descriptions of each dish, making sure to pronounce every word correctly.

Since my shrimp appetizer was the first dish to be served, my team and I took our places at the flattop. I could hear TJ announcing the first dish. His carefully enunciated description was met with a low rumble of approval from the diners, who were already enjoying sips of wine and last-minute, complimentary champagne cocktails.

Two doors connected the small, L-shaped dining room and the narrow kitchen; one opened onto the front half of the restaurant and one onto the back. In most areas of the kitchen, only one person could pass at a time, so our servers opted to line up single-file at each door, waiting for the kitchen crew to pass them the plates they would be serving. Those experienced in waiting tables carried four plates at a time; others could take only two. Only the sheer number of volunteer waitstaff got those plates to the tables as fast as they did, which was as soon as they were plated. The volunteers had been meticulously organized. Each was assigned two tables for which they would be responsible. Those servers would not only make sure the diners got their food but also explain the dishes, chat them up, and encourage them to hit the auction table.

Two other volunteers were assigned as "floaters." They drifted through the dining room, handing out ballots with each course. Doug, Leigh's husband, was responsible for tallying the votes. He took his place in the broom closet on the edge of the dining room. With a legal pad perched on an upside-down bucket, he worked his numerical magic. Our guests would assign each dish a score of one to five in each of three categories: originality, flavor, and plating.

In the kitchen, after dozens of dry runs of each plate, my team was so prepared for the way the dishes would be completed that we did not need to speak to one another. Our communication happened mostly in the form of head tilts and sideways glances. I demonstrated one plate, and my team took over the rest. Our human assembly line moved with mind-boggling efficiency and accuracy.

TJ rang the symbolic bell announcing the start of the dinner. Course number one—*go!* We all sprang into action. The steadiness of my voice surprised me as I called out the plating order to my line cooks: hot tortilla, seared shrimp, fried shrimp, salsa, sauce number one, sauce number two, tortilla strips. Our volunteers from the dining room yelled out what they needed, and we frantically filled the orders.

"I got a four-top. . . . No, sorry, make it five."

"Twofer here—I need two plates, now."

"Give me ten—ten plates, guys! That table has been waiting too long!"

We just kept going. No one looked up. No one wandered around aimlessly. All heads were down as fingers and hands chopped, placed, repositioned, garnished, and wiped.

At last, the words we had been waiting for: "That's it! Last table has their shrimp!" In unison, we dropped our tongs and spoons and shuffled out of Tom and his team's way. They were up and had only minutes to get their appetizer out. Even though our guests felt as if they got a brief break between courses, we in the kitchen did not pause for even a moment.

Tom's first course was to be a seared risotto cake with wild mushrooms and flakes of crispy pancetta. It was clear right away that their dish was not going out as fast as ours. Apparently, they had not gathered every Saturday and Sunday over the last six weeks, trying, timing, photographing, and trying again. As I stirred and tasted my soup, getting ready for the next course, I heard Chris. He had left his post as "schmoozer" with the guests and had come into the kitchen. His laugh was unmistakable. He took one look at the chaotic plating line on Tom's side and did exactly what anyone who knew him would have expected him to: he rolled up his sleeves and grabbed a plate.

"What are you *doing*?" I asked, half sputtering and half smiling. Of course, I knew exactly what he was doing—it was what he did best. Chris was coming to the rescue.

"Uh, I'm helping Tom get his appetizer out so that people aren't eating until midnight." He winked at me, challenging me to argue.

My Moroccan carrot soup was hot, and its flavor profile was optimal. The garnishes were ready, and Arlen and James were all over the prep for the salad, which would go out after the soup. So I did the natural thing: I jumped over to Tom's side and took my place next to Chris.

As I did in all aspects of my life, from disciplining our kids to rewarding my employees, I took my cue from him. "All right, Thomas! Show me how this slop of yours needs to be plated!" I called.

Tom shook his head, but he was undeniably relieved. As we plated and passed the plates to the servers, Chris edged closer to me and gave my hip a tap with his. With that small, playful gesture, he was telling me he was proud of me. Precisely at that moment, Rebekah Ulmer, our volunteer photographer, appeared. Despite the heat and humidity of the kitchen, Rebekah's blond hair was impeccably coiffed. Her flushed cheeks anchored the widest, brightest smile I had ever seen. I had known her for only a few months, but she had quickly made an indelible mark on my life. At the time of the food fight, my fondness for her was based on two things: her dry, edgy sense of humor (I nearly spit out my coffee during our first meeting) and her ability to produce a food mill in a pinch. Having realized the night before the food fight that I had to mill fifty pounds of potatoes and that I had only one food mill, I had put a call out for loaner mills. Within hours, Rebekah had produced one.

I would have no idea what a talented photographer she was until weeks after the food fight, when I finally had a chance to spend hours poring over the hundreds of beautiful pictures she had taken of everything and everyone to do with that memorable night. Now, as Chris and I worked on plating Tom's dish, Rebekah seemed to appear out of nowhere and snapped what would become one of my most cherished pictures of Chris and me. We had instinctively tilted our heads toward each other with a comfort only twenty years could have built. In that picture, Rebekah captured the simple secret of our happy marriage: friendship. My

face was devoid of makeup, and my crazy hair was hidden under a baseball cap embroidered with a pink breast cancer ribbon.
Chris had the slightest dark circles under his eyes, but his smile
was as natural as his jovial demeanor.

Not only did Chris begin helping instantly, but his presence
brought levity to the kitchen. Within moments of assuming his
place on Tom's line, he announced to everyone that he was an expert in restaurant kitchen work because, for the last seven years,
every night before bed he had been forced to watch past seasons of *Top Chef.* "Listen up, people! Here is what you all need
to know in order to keep this kitchen humming!" Most people
paused to hear this proclamation.

"You need to drop *f*-bombs—often. That's what they do. You
are not a real kitchen crew unless you have a foul mouth. Now
pass me that fucking pancetta."

I was known to curse around the house and our kids, but
Chris was much more reserved. The parade of filthy language
coming from his mouth was so unnatural, it was hilarious.
Through the laughter and energy of the kitchen, Rebekah floated, a barely noticeable figure, capturing countless indescribable
moments. She was so entrenched that her photos captured every
bit of agony, ecstasy, genius, and near disaster—wordlessly. Not
one of us watching her that night could ever have imagined that
in less than six months, Rebekah Ulmer would suffer from a sudden stroke that would leave the thirty-eight-year-old mother of
three fighting for her life.

Sometime around the soup course, Tom was ready to put
his rolled porchetta roast into the oven. It was a massive piece of
pork belly with the skin attached. Tom had stuffed and rolled it

and then tied it up with kitchen twine. As his team carried the huge trays of meat into the kitchen from the refrigerators, there was the slightest pause in the frenetic action—almost as if we all collectively held our breath.

At first, the roasts looked like amputated human legs. As the trays got closer, I noticed that the surface of the roasts was not smooth but rather appeared to be . . . bumpy? It wasn't until Tom's star protein was right next to me that those bumps became identifiable: they were nipples. The pork belly had been rolled such that row after row of pig teats was on the surface. Pig nipples. Dozens of them. Right before our eyes. I could think of nothing less appetizing. It was then that I got my second wind. There was no way I was going to lose to soft-core pig pornography.

The plan was for Tom to roast the pork belly and then use Pauly's meat slicer to portion it into thin discs. Because of the sheer size of the roasts and the thickness of the nipply skin, it would take a long time in a very hot oven to cook them properly. Tom had scooted me out of the way to bend down and put his roasts in the oven. As he shut the door and walked away, I noticed something. For the last twenty minutes, I had been standing just inches from a commercial-grade oven that had been preheated to four hundred degrees . . . and my legs were not getting hot. As the door opened, no blast of heat forced me back. Tom was too busy to notice. Without moving too much, so as not to attract attention to myself, I pulled open the oven door and stuck my hand in. The oven and Tom's pig nipples were ice cold. I was nothing short of gleeful as I anticipated my victory. Cooked nipples were going to be a tough sell; raw nipples were going to tip the scale my way for sure.

My joy lasted only a moment, though, before a raw and un-remitting feeling of guilt replaced it. I couldn't do it—I couldn't let him lose without even serving his signature dish. That victory for me would have been empty.

"Tom!" I yelled, not trying to hide the urgency in my voice. "Your oven's not hot—at all. Hope you have a plan B, friend."

Tom raced across the kitchen. He swatted at the beads of sweat on his red forehead with a dirty kitchen towel. "*Shit!*" His voice boomed, and his profanity had none of the humor in it that Chris's had.

We all scrambled around. "Someone get Pauly!" Our gracious host was serving as a guest judge and was sitting in the dining room, thoroughly enjoying the novelty of having someone cook for him.

Tom was coming out of the storage room in the kitchen. "Pizza ovens!" he called triumphantly, his face flushed with un-deniable relief.

Sure enough, tucked away from the main cooking area was a huge, state-of-the-art pizza oven. It could get really hot really fast and would quite possibly save Tom's entrée.

As Tom's main dish finally got cooking, my fluent team began to stutter. While the salads were coming together, I noticed an edginess in my crew. It seemed to me that they all knew something I didn't know. Finally, Arlen spoke. "Uh, Christine? We have a . . . uh . . . small problem."

Days before, I had gathered four teammates to help me coat balls of goat cheese with panko bread crumbs. The crispy-on-the-outside, gooey-on-the-inside goat cheese rounds were the star of the salad.

"We seem to be running out of cheese," Arlen said softly.
"That's not possible. We counted them; we counted one hundred and fifty goat cheese balls!" I whined. Then I realized "we" hadn't counted the balls at all. I had left this seemingly minor task to my twelve-year-old daughter and her two besties. Sometime that night, as their conversation turned to music and "pretty boys," a cheese ball or two must have been counted twice. It didn't matter what we had counted or, as was becoming obvious, miscounted—we were not going to have enough cheese for all of the plates. That could be a fatal error. We had no time to buy, roll, coat, and fry more goat cheese.

The stress in the kitchen was peaking. James, my sous chef, broke my temporary paralysis: "We have some left! If we cut them in half, we'll make it!" And then Tom followed up with the ideal response: "Perfect. Come on, guys—everybody *cut the cheese!*"

Just as the laughter was dying down, Doug joined us. He had left his post in the broom closet to bring important news. Several guests had asked for beer. When they'd learned that for the charity event we were serving only wine, some had become irritable and left. Those guests storming out were not the biggest news, however. It turned out that they had gone only to return a few minutes later with several cases of beer. As they'd drunk it, they'd grown more and more rowdy and were now beginning to upset other guests.

Doug read the panic on my face. "Don't worry, C—we have it under control out there. I just wanted to keep you up to speed." As he turned and walked away, Doug called, "Oh, and by the way, with the entrées about to go out, he has you by about thirty points." Despite Tom's team's seeming lack of organization and his dwindling confidence, he was managing to put out really tasty plates.

My mouth suddenly felt dry. I knew that Doug, who had developed a firm yet gentle method of discipline in his job as a second-grade teacher, would easily defuse the rambunctious crowd.

It took only a few minutes for my confidence to be restored. As my braised short rib plates began coming back into the kitchen after they'd been cleared, everyone noticed something: they had all been practically licked clean. Tom's pork plates, however, often returned untouched. He was staggering on the heels of the pig nipples. One solid punch with my dessert, and it would be all over.

As painstaking as the making of the ice cream had been, the plating was more so. We had rimmed miniature martini glasses half with sugar and half with salt. Then we topped each scoop of ice cream with hand-dipped chocolate-covered pretzels and garnished it with a sliver of "sugar glass." We had made the clear amber candy days ahead by pouring scalding melted sugar onto a sheet pan. Once the molten sugar had solidified, we had shattered the sheets one by one by sealing them in Ziploc bags and throwing them, with a great deal of ceremony, on my ceramic kitchen floor.

I stood at the end of the dessert assembly line, inspecting every single dish of ice cream before it went out. "More pretzels!" "Where's the sugar?" "This one's not rimmed!" Exhaustion was making me a bit snippy. So it was with an audible sigh of relief that the kitchen team broke into applause as the emcee rang the bell that officially brought the contest to an end.

Tom and Chris surrounded me and squeezed me in a massive three-person hug. I wiped my face on my apron and hugged my team. Then it was time. A winner was about to be announced.

Despite the almost-unbearable heat of the kitchen, my hands were ice cold and my heart pounded against my chest wall. Although I had told myself for weeks that winning and losing did not matter, there was only one way to explain the feeling in my gut: I wanted to win—badly. After Tom and I each spoke to our guests, our two local celebrity judges critiqued each dish. The intimidating panel of judges was still blind as to who had made what.

Pauly and Adrian Martinez, a well-known local artist whose work could be found in the White House, were our judges, and they were not exactly gentle in their critiques.

"No idea what that tortilla was doing on that plate. Totally not necessary—and so dry!"

I felt myself cringe.

"Loved both soups, but that carrot soup, while flavorful, was a bit . . . how do I say? Pedestrian?"

As they worked their way to the entrées, I braced myself. For the third time that night, Tom put his arm around me. I wrapped an exhausted arm around his waist and rested my head against his chest.

"The sauce on the pork dish was delicious, but really, the meat was just too fatty and underdone. Now, about those short ribs . . ."

I held my breath. The diners' votes were being tallied, but in my gut I knew that whichever direction the judges went, the guests would have followed.

Pauly went first. He shook his head as he looked down at his notes.

"Well, I could just have taken a bath in those short ribs. Unbelievable. Only thing better all night was that salted-caramel ice cream."

With that, my team was around me, hugging and high-fiving. As I tried to break free from their enthusiastic embrace, I scanned the room for Chris. He was leaning against the back wall of the kitchen, twisting a dirty kitchen towel in his hands. Our eyes locked, and in that moment I knew I would be victorious. I hadn't officially won, but Chris had that look—the same look he had given me in the delivery room when Hadley was born and on that steamy day when he dragged me out on my first run.

My team stood in a semicircle in the middle of the hushed crowd, our arms linked together, as TJ spoke. He began by announcing, "Risotto cakes, crab bisque, warm mushroom salad, porchetta, and goat cheese pudding belong to . . . Chef Tom!" There was a burst of applause, cheering, and whistling. Someone yelled out, "Yeah, Tommy! Knew you'd show that little girl who's boss!" The applause seemed to last a really long time.

TJ continued, as he pulled me gently to his side, "That can mean only that this little lady is responsible for the shrimp *taquitos*, Moroccan carrot soup, baby arugula salad, braised short ribs, and salted-caramel ice cream!" The applause for me was just as loud and enthusiastic. Doug handed TJ the envelope with the final tally in it.

"Well. Isn't this interesting?" he began. The next seconds felt like an eternity. I glanced around the room at our sated and happy guests and marveled at what my team had accomplished in that one night. Over forty strangers gathered on February 23, 2013. They introduced themselves to one another and shared how they had come to the team. As they folded napkins and polished glasses, they told their cancer stories. The evening wore on as these strangers and our guests celebrated having waged courageous cancer battles all around. They cried for the lives lost and cheered for the survivors seated in our midst.

At the start of the evening, I had choked back tears as I gave my short welcome speech. Now, waiting for the verdict, I once again scanned the room, catching my sister's eye and warm smile. Tears spilled. At the table across from her sat Linda Hall. When I spotted my longtime patient, my quiet tears turned to guttural sobs. Linda had come to see me several years before with "digestive issues." She really just wanted advice on diet changes so that she could manage her bloating. It took a few visits, but finally I was able to convince her that she needed an abdominal ultrasound. In my mind, Linda's worst-case scenario was that she would need to have her gallbladder removed. The ultrasound showed a completely normal gallbladder but a hideous ovarian tumor. Linda would have died of her Stage III ovarian cancer, but there she sat. She had survived surgery, chemo, and radiation. Most important, she had lived to see her oldest daughter get married. Over the years, Linda kept trying to credit me with saving her life. The reality is that ovarian cancer was nowhere on my radar. What saved Linda's life was her trust in my judgment. That trust was what led her to the ultrasound, oncologist, and surgeon and ultimately to her seat as our honored guest.

I thought of the imaginary food fight trophy and of Linda's and Debi's and Joe's trust in me. It was a trust placed around my neck like a race medal—one that weighed a hundred pounds. I was proud to have earned it and yet at times felt unbearably burdened by it. I craved this "light" food fight trophy, which could be mine without the burdens of those trusting yet dying patients.

TJ's voice brought me back to the final moment of the long contest between Tom and me. "By the end of the salad course, these chefs were neck and neck. *But*, with a margin of just twenty-eight points out of a possible total of nearly eight thousand, the winner is . . ."

I don't remember hearing my name. I just remember Tom's lifting me off my feet and twirling me around and around as I cried. Just as he set me down, Chris was in front of me, and he, too, hugged me and picked me up. "I am so proud of you, babe!" he whispered in my ear. While there was no tangible prize, Chris was congratulating me on the enormity of our accomplishment. When all was said and done, in three hours, forty-some strangers had served 104 diners not one, but two, five-course meals. In that one night, we had plated, presented, and cleared 1,040 plates of food.

But as I reveled in my victory, little did I know that hundreds of miles away, outside Boston, two brothers were plotting a vicious attack—one that, in forty-nine days, would threaten to destroy everything our team had worked so hard to accomplish.

Chapter 10: Is There a Doctor on Board?

If you want to go fast, go alone. If you want to go far, go together.

—African proverb

It was midnight, the place was clearing out, and the volunteer dishwashers were soaked from head to toe. The waitstaff's fatigue had caused them to become careless when loading dirty plates onto trays. The kitchen floor was covered in water, and the trays were brutally heavy. As we all were laughing, giddy from our event, and wiping sleep from our eyes, a massive, full tray of rented dishes slipped out of a volunteer's hands and crashed to the floor with a sickening shatter.

There was a split-second pause as everyone caught their breath. Then Chris broke the silence. "Oh, hey—no worries!" He slapped Mike, the mortified dishwasher, on the back and bent to pick up shards of china and glass. "Aw, it's just dishes. Don't worry about it, man. . . . I'm sure my wife will find a way of guilting the rental company into 'donating' them." Everyone laughed as, once again, nearly unbearable tension dissipated.

When the last piece of broken glass had been swept up and the sopping floors had been polished, we all collapsed in booths around the dining room and reveled in the magnitude of our accomplishment. By the end of the night, our shirts were filthy and wet, but no one seemed to be in any hurry to get them off. Booth after booth was filled with people half lying and half sitting. Wendy Ford, whose mother had beaten cancer seven times, had her head on another girl's shoulder. Someone was helping Amy, my nurse practitioner and Tom's wife, carry auction debris to her car. As I watched them walk out the door, my heart filled with admiration at how far all of these people had come. This night and this event had done that. They had turned strangers into friends with an unbreakable bond.

TJ sat on the floor with his back against a wall as his wife, Maria, laid her head on his shoulder.

Out of the blue, someone called out, "Hey! Is anyone else . . . hungry?" Laughter erupted. For as much food as we had served to all of our paying guests, our volunteers had gotten not one morsel, and it had been hours since their simple meal of pizza and beer. I visualized every empty and scrubbed clean pot in the kitchen. There was nothing left to offer my friends. Then it came to me: we did have plenty of leftover ice cream. I ran to the back freezer and emerged with an armful of quart-size containers of my winning dessert. Tom jumped up and grabbed fistfuls of spoons from the drawers. Groups of three or four people huddled around each quart. The spoons were still hot from the dishwasher and melted right into the luscious ice cream. Everyone's eyes closed, and they all uttered grunts of approval. I sat wedged between Tom, my competitor, and Chris, my best friend and life partner. I doubted that anything could ever feel so good or so right as that moment.

Sometime around 2:30 in the morning, the door opened and we all sprang to attention. Pauly was back. *What is he doing here? Oh God. Did we clean the bathrooms? Did someone remember to scrub the flattop?* As my panicked thoughts raced through my foggy mind, Pauly smiled. He looked sickeningly refreshed. He was clean-shaven, save for the thin, well-maintained strip of hair around his chin. His shirt was clean and pressed and tucked into jeans. Just hours before, he had been in the dining room, dressed in khakis and a sport coat.

"Good morning, y'all!" Pauly called jovially.

Good morning? I must be dreaming. I haven't been to bed in nearly two days!

Pauly must have seen the confusion on our faces. He pulled a clean white apron from the closet behind the bar. As he quickly tied it around his waist, he explained, "I got my breakfast business showing up in a few hours. It's time to make the scones!"

Pauly's café was famous for his scones. The flavors just came to him, and he ran with them. My favorite was the white chocolate–cherry flavor. The scones were crumbly and not too sweet. They were also about the size of a baby's head. I always told myself that I couldn't possibly eat a whole one, but then I somehow managed to. Pauly was funny and brilliant about his scones. Every morning, he made a fixed number. When those scones ran out, that was it for the day. Sometimes they would be gone before

9:00 A.M. I once asked him about it. "Why don't you just make more the next week? You're losing money every week, aren't you?"

"Nope," he explained. "These scones are legendary. People just come the next week and bring their friends. Or they order a dozen for their brunch party. Having them just out of reach makes people want 'em that much more!"

"Anyone in the mood to help me in the kitchen?" Pauly was asking now.

At any other moment, I would have jumped at the chance to make Pauly's famous scones with him, but right then I was contemplating asking Chris and Tom to carry me out of the place. The thought of cooking or baking anything made me want to cry. Clearly, I was not alone. After a flurry of mumbled excuses, the booths began to clear out. Not one person jumped up. People creaked, leaned, moaned, and shuffled as they headed out into the cold, starless night. The sun wouldn't be up for a few hours, and while Pauly was making his scones, I would get the best five hours of sleep I had had in weeks.

Sometime around 8:00 A.M., I woke up feeling surprisingly refreshed . . . and starving. I winced as I rolled over onto my right side and felt the massive bruise there. Then I giggled as I recalled how I had gotten it. In my racing from kitchen to dining room and back, I had barreled directly into the corner of one of the dining tables, hip-first.

I smelled the coffee before I saw it. Steam rose from my favorite, huge glass mug, which Chris had set carefully on my nightstand. He knew that I would need at least a few sips before I attempted to put my swollen feet on the floor.

I was a good bit through my coffee, to which Chris had added the right amount of cream and just a touch of sugar, when Hadley came skipping into my room. As she scrambled up onto my bed, I lifted the mug off my lap to keep it from spilling. She was fully dressed in skintight black jeans, a black leather jacket, and pink cowboy boots. I didn't care that half of her outfit had been, at least at one point, part of a Halloween costume.

"Mommy! I'm *hungry!*"

Chris was a few steps behind her. "You hungry, Mama?" He smiled.

"Sure am! What are you in the mood for?" I peered at my little girl's adorable face, thankful for the promise of a Sunday full of time with her, Maisy, Sam, and Chris. I felt like I had been away for months.

"Scones!" Hadley called.

We looked at each other and laughed. We were not getting away from Pauly's scones that day, no matter what.

I stood under a scalding-hot shower and let the water just run over me. Various open wounds, scrapes, and burns screamed in protest. I washed my hair but didn't bother with the three different products I typically applied. Instead, I twisted the lot of it into a wet bun, which I pulled through the back of my now-famous pink baseball cap. Yoga pants and a cotton T-shirt rounded out my outfit. I took the stairs slowly, stopping for a second on each one to allow my burning thighs to recover. Once at the bottom, I realized that I had forgotten shoes, but the staircase looked as intimidating as Mount Everest, so I slipped my still-swollen feet into a pair of Ugg slippers lying in the laundry room.

Chris already had the kids in the car. As I hobbled out of the house and into the driveway, he jumped out and came around to help me into the passenger seat of his huge truck. I literally could not lift my leg that high without holding on to him.

"You okay there, old lady? Good thing you have a few weeks to get ready for that ten-mile run!"

It hadn't even occurred to me that the food fight prep had really stymied my running. I would have to get back on track. But not till tomorrow.

When we got to the Blue Cafe and sat down, Patti, Pauly's wife and business partner, came to our table. I jumped up and threw my arms around her. "Thank you so much, Patti."

She patted me on the back and pushed me back into my chair. "Honey, you look like you haven't had a decent meal in days! Pauly will whip you up something to fill that little stomach of yours! You deserve to have somebody cook for *you* now!"

I ate my three-egg omelet with mushrooms and peppers, crisp hash browns, and buttery toast in minutes. The kids poked at each other over their scones and pancakes, and Chris sipped his coffee quietly. Every few minutes, he looked up over his Sunday paper and smiled at me. When he said, "Want something else to eat, fatty? I can ask Pauly if he has a cow back there," I knew what he meant.

Translation: *I am so glad to see you eating. I love you, and I am so very proud of you.*

* * *

That night, I did the math. After expenses, the food fight had netted our team nearly $9,000. When the evening began, we had already raised over $25,000. I felt my heart fill as I recalled our initial goal to raise a mere $2,000. If we, as a team, just shut down at that moment and did not raise another cent, we would still have broken countless fund-raising records. But of course I knew the team wouldn't stop. I wouldn't let them, and they wouldn't let me.

Knowing that we had met and exceeded every goal I had set was a wonderful send-off for our much-anticipated spring break trip to Sedona, Arizona. It didn't really matter if the team did anything in terms of fund-raising during this vacation; as I boarded the flight, I mentally cut myself loose. I vowed to make the next ten days about one thing and one thing only: my family. Until my feet hit the ground in Philadelphia again, I was not going to be a runner, a chef, a team captain, or a doctor. It turned out, I was off in my declaration by only a few hours, as I would be forced to put my doctor hat on a bit before we returned to Philadelphia soil.

Our spring break trip was like a honeymoon for our family. The team, the food fight, and my devastatingly sick patients had taken up every free minute of my time. My kids and husband missed having me around. And so, together, over ten days, we hiked amazing terrain, relaxed under the bluest of skies, and let the warm sun melt away the stress of recent weeks. After that blissful interlude, it was with a heavy heart that I lugged my children and our hastily packed luggage through the Phoenix airport and to the dreaded security line.

As we waited for our stuff at the end of the line, I was so consumed with keeping my eyes fixed on my favorite bracelets, which I had been forced to put in a plastic bowl, and on Hadley's favorite blankie that I failed to notice that our hastily packed carry-on full of wet, stinky shoes and a few toiletries was getting a lot of attention from a buxom TSA agent. Sure enough, the worker—wearing the finest blue forensic gloves—pulled our family aside. In much the same way as I had, years before, as a surgery student, extracted a festering and forgotten sponge from a patient's reopened abdominal cavity, Agent Morris extracted a leaking Ziploc bag from the outer pocket of the shoe suitcase, containing Dove Body Wash, Suave Detangling Spray, and a still-full bottle of NO-AD sunscreen. I shrugged off the loss of the toiletries as I glanced at my watch. Our flight home would board in twenty minutes. We reassembled our ravaged carry-ons and made sure everyone had their precious items. It would be a six-hour flight home, so we stocked up on snacks and water. Everyone but me chose a bit of easy reading material. I planned on spending the entire duration of the flight answering the hundreds of e-mails I was sure were awaiting me.

Finally, we were on the plane and everyone was settled with snacks, books, and devices. Five-year-old Hadley was already whining.

"No, Haddie, you cannot watch *Brave* until the pilot says it's okay. . . . Because he is the pilot, and he is in charge of everything that happens on this plane."

At thirty thousand feet, I had spent my $14 on in-flight Internet and was knee-deep in various e-mails when the intercom crackled to life. A slightly panic-stricken flight attendant came on, asking for a doctor or nurse or "any medical person" to step forward.

Instinct beat rational thinking as my hand went up. Moments later, I was ushered to the front of the plane, where lay an ashen woman.

"This is Grace," one of the flight attendants announced. Grace was wearing an oxygen mask. Someone thrust a sphygmomanometer into my hand. The state-of-the-art blood pressure cuff had obviously never been used. It was still encased in plastic.

I pulled the cuff out of its packaging and began firing off questions. The elderly woman had stood up, felt dizzy and nauseous, and fainted. I called for someone to get a list of any medications she might have taken. I was rewarded with a large Ziploc bag full of blood pressure and cardiac medications. Flight attendants buzzed around with useless information. I nodded absentmindedly as my heart sank right along with the mercury on the sphygmomanometer.

58/40.

I released the valve, then pumped up the cuff again. It had to be a mistake.

56/42.

It was not a mistake. The lady at my feet barely had a blood pressure. Unless that changed, and quickly, she was going to die.

I heard my voice ask for an emergency kit.

My pleading eyes were met with blank stares from four flight attendants.

"You know, IVs, medicine, a defibrillator—anything?"

Finally, someone moved. A giant black bag landed on the floor next to my feet, along with the sweetest words out of the mouth of an angel: "Doc, I'm Jackie, and I'm an ER nurse. Can I help you?"

Inside my brain, I yelled, *Hell yeah! Thank God!* It had been nearly twenty years since I had successfully placed an IV in a dying patient. I thought of Debi and my failed attempt at placing her IV. Then I remembered how I had learned to do IVs in the first place. I was a med student then, on the IV team in the hospital. When I first took the overnight shift, it was to make extra money for books. I did eventually get good at IVs, but the veteran nurse manager was right all those years ago. I had overheard her grumbling in the break room, "Why do those medical students think that just because they're going to be doctors, they can place IVs? I wish they would just stick to the books and leave the IVs to me. I do not have time to be cleaning up after these kids all night long!" It was true then and truer now. I had *no* business inserting the IV line Grace crucially needed into her arm.

My voice sounded steady as I responded to Jackie. "Sure, thanks. How about putting a twenty-gauge in Grace's AC vein so we can give her some fluids and a blood pressure?" Jackie did not need translation. She knew that meant I was asking her to place the largest-bore IV possible in the crook of Grace's arm, also known as the antecubital space, in order for us to administer some normal saline. I prayed that the saline would help Grace's blood pressure to recover.

We got to work, Jackie and I. We had never laid eyes on each other but moved in such harmony, it seemed as if we had worked together a lifetime. We hoped that we could at least buy time by correcting Grace's low blood pressure via administering IV saline. I heard Jackie calling for the IV connector and looked down to see that she had already successfully placed the IV line—she had done it in seconds and without a single drop of Grace's blood anywhere to show for it. This was a sharp contrast with my early attempts at IV placement. Once, an overnight janitor came into one of my patient's rooms after I had successfully placed an IV in an elderly patient. The old man shook his head as he reached for gloves. "Mm-mm-mm. What in the Lord's name did you do in here, child? Surgery?" I had made a mental note to clean up the hemorrhage next time.

Once Grace's IV was in place, we ran fluids, measured her blood pressure, and rifled through her bag of medicines, frantically looking for any possible clues about her condition. Was she diabetic? Did she have heart disease? Had she become confused and begun taking the wrong combination of pills?

70/50.

Color was returning to Grace's face, but her cool, clammy skin made my stomach clench; I knew that meant she was still in danger. As sweat saturated my T-shirt and frizzed the hair at my temples, the cockpit door opened. It was then that my eyes met with the shiniest, nicest pair of loafers I had ever seen a man wear. Captain Atkins was exactly what you would imagine a pilot to be: tall, tan, handsome, composed, and completely clueless about the goings-on at his feet. I thought of my reprimand to Hadley just hours before. "The pilot is in charge of everything on this plane!" Yeah. Not so much the medical disasters, though.

"So," he began. "I understand we have a situation here. I am going to use this lavatory, and then I would like the details."

With that, he stepped over our laid-out patient, barely missing my outstretched hand holding the IV line in place. Jackie and I exchanged a knowing look.

Moments later, he reappeared. As he adjusted the buckle on his black belt, he seemed to be illustrating just how relieved his bladder was. Now Captain Atkins was ready for the scoop.

Thankfully, Jackie spoke for me. She explained Grace's medical status slowly and clearly. As the pilot blinked blankly, I felt my blood begin to boil.

The tower had been notified. They had contacted their physician liaisons on the ground. Per protocol, our patient had to achieve and maintain a blood pressure no lower than 90/60, or our fearless leader was going to have to divert the plane to St. Louis.

"Ninety over sixty, girls. That's the magic number. Get me that number, and I will get us all home on time."

Whew. Thank God I have some incentive now. I was going to let Grace die, but I really did want to get home on time. . . . St. Louis really would mess me up, I thought.

Jackie and I waited until Captain Suave was back in his cockpit. We knew what we had to do. We had to get Grace's blood pressure up to 90/60 and keep it there. For hours, we squeezed the bags of saline. We attempted to achieve reverse Trendelenburg. This medical technique of lowering a patient's head while raising her legs helps to get blood to the brain. In ERs and hospitals, this is accomplished by pushing a lever that lowers the head of an automated mattress. On flight 964, we commandeered every pillow, blanket, and sweatshirt to raise Grace's legs. At one point, an off-duty police officer offered to hold our patient's legs up in the air for us. At the sight of the well-built man holding our pale patient's legs like the arms of a wheelbarrow, I almost cried. That position stripped poor Grace of her dignity, and besides, it put too much pressure on her neck, so we were soon back to the blankets.

I felt a small tap on my shoulder and turned around to see Hadley clutching her blankie. Wordlessly, she offered it to me— her most treasured possession of her five years on Earth. "Mom, look!" Hadley pointed to her middle name—Grace—embroidered in pink satin. I did cry then. I hugged her and shooed her back down the aisle to her dad.

Finally, we had it: 92/60. Grace even smiled once or twice. We all breathed sighs of relief. Well, that is, until I realized that for the entire three hours, my back had been facing the main cabin—in a squatting position—in my favorite low-rise jeans. My assuagement at Grace's improvement was squelched by the realization that I had exposed my very own plumber's butt to all of those people sitting in coach.

Despite her improvement, Grace was still not stable. Jackie and I were afraid to move because every time we raised her head a few inches or repositioned her in any way, her blood pressure dropped. We pulled the head flight attendant aside and in urgent, hushed tones asked how quickly we could land in St. Louis.

"Uh, St. Louis, honey? We missed that window hours ago. We're going to Philly!"

Shit.

"How long till we land?" I stammered. By that point, I could not feel my toes and my bladder was the size of Texas.

One hour till Philly airspace. Four and a half hours had passed in a blink.

Jackie and I huddled and talked and figured that the best plan was just to hold steady until we landed. We were not moving our patient—no matter what—until we landed.

Think again.

Captain Atkins was out again. He smiled. His second-in-command was flying the plane while the captain sparkled white veneers at us.

"Nice work, ladies. Now, we are going to need to get this young lady into a seat, with her seat belt fastened for landing."

In one voice, Jackie and I emphatically shouted, "No way!"

Jackie followed up in her best soothing voice, not at all like my irate, wanna-kick-him-in the-face tone: "Sir, we absolutely cannot move this patient. If we do, her blood pressure will plummet."

Captain Atkins stood up and cracked his sore back. After all, he had been crouching for an entire thirty seconds. He looked pensive for a moment.

"I don't want to influence your care, Doctor, but in order to land this plane, I need this lady in a seat with her seat belt fastened."

"Well, sir, I guess we'd all better get used to cruising at thirty thousand feet, because *there is no way in hell you are going to get Grace—she has a name—in a seat with her goddamn seat belt fastened without killing her!*"

A well-meaning flight attendant chose this moment to chime in. "Couldn't you give her CPR or something?"

In a barely controlled whisper, I responded with feigned patience, "Um, well, generally we don't like to give CPR to patients who are awake—but thanks for your suggestion."

By now, Jackie and I no longer needed to speak; we just used our eyes to communicate. I felt intimidated by this tall, uniformed man standing over me, so I chose to stand, too. Without giving any thought to decorum or appearance, I pulled my panties out of my ass, hoisted my waistband over my crack, and tugged my shirt down in the back. I blew a hopeless wisp of hair out of my right eye and spoke. "Explain to me what happens in a situation where it is just not feasible or safe to put a passenger in a seat for landing."

Captain Atkins was so somber, I expected him to say something catastrophic, like, *Well, we fly around until we run out of gas and then fall out of the sky to meet our fate—a fate we deserve, at that, for not having everyone in a seat with their seat belt fastened.*

"Well . . ." He spoke in the tone of someone addressing a two-year-old. "We need to declare an emergency."

Wordlessly, my eyes questioned, *And?*

"And, well, that means *a lot* of paperwork for me."

Welcome to my world, Captain Atkins. Need a pen?

We secured our patient in the first-class aisle. Jackie and I sat in our seats, with our seat belts fastened, and leaned over, monitoring Grace closely and periodically checking her vital signs and responsiveness. We cooed and stroked her forehead. Our backs screamed and our heads throbbed, but we smiled and reassured her she was going to be just fine.

Finally, we felt the rumble of the Philly asphalt beneath us.

I had never been more relieved than I was at that moment to see the flashing lights of the ambulance waiting by the Jetway. Once the EMTs were aboard, I got up slowly and headed back to my seat. Just as I crossed into coach, I was stunned to hear the entire cabin erupt in applause and high fives. Despite the raucous cheering, I heard, from way in the back, a distinctive "Way to go, Mom."

Something changed in me on that flight. I suddenly felt empowered, smart, and useful again. I felt my self-esteem push back against the months of battering I had given it. Ironically, after a ten-day vacation in one of the most beautiful places in the world, I experienced all of my real restoration during the harrowing five-and-a-half-hour flight home.

* * *

Over the next several weeks, Team CMMD got back to its to-gether-but-separate way of gathering exclusively on Facebook. We cheered each other on as our dollars ticked up. By early April, we had raised over $40,000. We were exactly one month from race day and were languishing in our accomplishments. No one felt it necessary to push harder on the fund-raising front, but, buoyed by the joyous time we'd had at the food fight, my new-found spunk, and a gorgeous spring forecast, we scheduled our first official "group run" for April 7, 2013.

Seventeen people showed up that day. Among them was a man named Earl. Earl was one of those guys I never would have met were it not for the team and for Facebook. While he was not a runner, he was a spirited supporter, always cheering for us from the sidelines, and he had become "one" of us. As the Broad Street Run drew near-er, I began planning our post-race party and was looking for a caterer to do a barbecue. Earl commented that he had just the guy. I was so thrilled to have a connection that I promised Earl an invitation to the team party—even though he wasn't really part of the team.

"Well, if I come to the party, I have to be on the team—officially," he said definitively.

I learned that when one runner dropped out of the team because of an injury, I would be able to substitute another. Before making it official, I sent Earl a Facebook message: "I can get you on the Broad Street Run team, Earl. But can you . . . run?"

Earl had in fact been running some as he trained for a 5K race, which, at 3.1 miles, was less than a third of the distance of the Broad Street Run—now just four weeks away. Earl agreed to join us on our first official group run that Sunday, April 7. We all needed to get in seven miles—and Earl had never run more than three.

That morning was cold, but everyone who had promised to show up was there. The seventeen of us bounced around, warming our muscles. There was only a split second of awkward silence when I yelled, "All right, ladies! Let's go!" Then, as the group of seventeen men and women fell in line behind me, I gradually picked up the pace from a slow jog to a brisker run, all the while keeping an eye on the back of the pack.

At the one-mile mark, clear distinctions in pace declared themselves. Arlen, my right-hand man in the kitchen, took off ahead of me with several runners, I held down the middle, and Earl and a couple of slower runners brought up the rear. As we ran, the sun poked through the clouds and the creek alongside us shimmered brightly. The endorphins, the camaraderie, and the sunshine came together to create an atmosphere of utter giddiness. We called out to random strangers, "Good morning!" We offered high fives to anyone coming from the other direction and practically ran frightened strangers off the trail.

Several miles into the run, Arlen and his fast runners reached the halfway mark and began turning around. As we slower runners identified the folks coming toward us as fellow teammates, we erupted in raucous applause. When I passed Arlen, he met my high five with such force, I thought he had dislocated my shoulder. And so it went, faster runners looping around to be congratulated by slower ones.

As we closed in on the last mile of our training run that morning, I looked back. I could not see Earl. Everyone else was accounted for. We all waited at the end of the trail, breathless and sweaty, peering down the path, hoping for any glimpse of our newest teammate.

Just as Arlen was getting ready to head down the trail in search of him, Earl's figure emerged—tiny and partially obscured by the bright haze of the sun. He was moving slowly, but he was still running. One other thing was painfully clear: Earl was alone. Before I could grasp what was happening, Arlen and the group of faster runners who had been the first to finish took off toward him, hooting and hollering all the way. When they reached him, those runners surrounded Earl like a group of fighter jets in formation. Earl was grinning, and he was running . . . fast. From that day on, it was a tradition for our team's faster runners to repeat legs of their training runs in order to meet up with and escort slower runners to the finish, so none of our runners ever finished a training run alone.

The next morning, Earl posted that he was barely able to walk. As was common practice by that point, his complaining post was met with a smattering of good advice to "drink lots of water," "eat a banana, and rest." Those nuggets of wisdom were eclipsed by an avalanche of comments like "What's the matter, Earl—you a *girl?*" and "C'mon, Earl, pull your panties up and move your slow ass." With that, Earl was officially a member of our team.

We had less than thirty days to go until race day, and our team energy exploded as Earl's inclusion rallied us in indescribable ways. Earl raised his required $500 just days after that group run. As his story filtered out through Facebook, our friends came to life. Many who had already donated did so again. In the nine days following Earl's first group run, we raised another $20,000.

We felt unstoppable—on the trail, in our fund-raising, and in our spirit.

Then, on April 15, 2013, just two weeks before the Philadelphia Broad Street Run, it all came crashing to a halt.

Chapter 11: FALLING DOWN

Thinking will not overcome fear, but action will.

—W. Clement Stone

That day started much like every Monday. I climbed into my car, balancing hot coffee, phone, and briefcase while fumbling through my purse for my perpetually missing keys. As I slid into the driver's seat, I winced. My quads screamed from my run the day before. It was such an odd—almost welcome—kind of pain, reminding me of my accomplishment. I giggled a little to myself as I remembered that crazy nine-miler.

My running music had always seemed to affect my speed—the zippier the tune, the faster I ran. Halfway through Sunday's run, as they struggled to keep up, my running mates asked what I was jamming to. My answer filtered down the trail, and one by one they all erupted in laughter. Some laughed so hard they had to stop to catch their breath. I was never going to live down my taste in running music. Apparently, Miley Cyrus's "Hoedown

Throwdown"—the line-dancing tune made famous by squealing tweens—did not have the same appeal to "serious" athletes as epic songs like "Eye of the Tiger."

Hot coffee, found keys, and good pain quickly gave way to late patients and prostate exams, and in a blink, the day was ending. I could not wait to get home.

I had promised Chris long ago, as part of my no-distracted-driving pledge, that I would not reach for my ringing, buzzing, dinging phone while in the car. In order to save myself from breaking my promise, I had taken to putting my phone inside my briefcase and putting the briefcase in the backseat. If it was out of reach, I wouldn't be tempted to go after it.

I had been on the road for less than a minute when my bag virtually came to life. With every consecutive ding, I felt my blood pressure rise and my driving focus fade. Finally, I couldn't take it anymore, and at the next red light, I broke down, groping around for my phone with the guilt and longing of an adulteress reaching for her forbidden lover.

Just this once. I'll just check it for a second. It might be the office. Did I forget Mrs. Cooperstein's laxative prescription? I'll put the phone away as soon as the light turns.

It took the car behind me several honks to get my attention. I was completely perplexed by the text on my screen. Was it a misfired message intended for someone else? Or was *I* missing something?

"What are you going to say to your team about Boston?"

That first message was from Danielle, my neighbor and a dear friend. It was followed by several more texts from all sorts of people asking me what I thought and how I felt and what I was going to do.

When I parked in my driveway, I realized that I was still clutching the phone and I couldn't remember how I'd gotten home. It was not possible to be more distracted than that. Something bad and big had happened in Boston, and it had something to do with Team CMMD, but I had no idea what, why, or how.

I cursed myself for never having gotten around to learning how to work the satellite radio in my car. Most days, my trips to and from the office were so short that I never even thought about the radio. But not on April 15—something newsworthy had happened, and I had missed it. I didn't bother to pull the car into the garage. I grabbed my bag, threw open the laundry room door, and bolted into the kitchen.

I gave Maisy and Sam each a quick peck on the cheek and then went about switching on every TV in the house. Each was tuned to a different news outlet. Each played the same horrifying images of amputated limbs, splintered bones, and splattered blood. At first I tried to shield my two older kids from the news, but, thanks to their mobile devices, they had both already heard about Boston hours before. Hadley was a different story. She was absolutely terrified of blood and gore. Naturally, her older siblings, during the rare times they paid her any attention, took great pleasure in exposing her to "severed limbs," complete with ketchup blood and feigned pain. She would not handle this grisly news well.

"Haddie!" I called, trying to sound chipper.

"Mommmmmmmy!" Hadley always greeted me as if I had been gone a month. I bent down and hugged her to me. She started to wriggle, reminding me that I was squeezing her too tightly for a normal day.

"How about an episode of *Good Luck Charlie* on the iPad?"

Her eyes widened. "Really? It's Monday!"

Chris was almost maniacal in his enforcement of our household's "no TV Monday through Friday" rule. It was ingrained in our kids. But this was not any ordinary Monday. I needed time to gather information and to think. Hadley's treat would buy me at least half an hour.

Over the afternoon, as the news filtered in, my hands grew increasingly colder and my stomach turned. There had been a bombing at the finish line of the Boston Marathon. Several people had been killed or critically injured. I watched with horror as the images unfolded, while I recalled the morning of September 11, 2001. My now-teen daughter had been in her high chair, eating Cheerios off a plastic tray one at a time, when our world had changed forever. This Monday afternoon, I had that same terrorizing feeling of utter powerlessness and dread. I couldn't shake the sense that our world just might be ending.

While a manhunt went on in Boston, I turned my mind to my team of forty-seven runners at home. What would they think? What would we do? Would the Philadelphia Broad Street Run be canceled? Would we be safe?

On Facebook, cover photos were changed to images of the Boston skyline. Profile pictures displayed symbolic red socks. Our country was, as it had twelve years before, rallying in the face of tragedy. But along with the symbolic patriotism, Facebook was disseminating a plethora of conspiracy theories. Most noticeable to me were the ones linking the Boston Marathon to the Philadelphia Broad Street Run. Both were historic city races. Both were widely publicized. And both drew tens of thousands of innocent bystanders to venues that were nearly impossible to keep secure.

While rumors circulated recklessly, it became clear that I needed to make some sort of rally call to my teammates. Our race was in less than three weeks. Most of my runners were leaner, faster, and happier than they had ever been. We had already broken every fund-raising record. With every mile we ran and every dollar we raised, we were honoring our loved ones. More importantly, we were healing our own broken spirits. To have accomplished so much and then not cross the finish line would be devastating to every runner on my team. I needed to be my team's cheerleader, captain, and voice of reassurance. There was just one problem with that: I was terrified. I was afraid of dying. I was afraid of leaving my kids motherless. I was afraid for my team.

So much so that for the first few hours after the news broke, I quietly prayed for the Broad Street Run to be canceled so the decision would no longer be mine to make. I paced around my bedroom, watching the news and stalking my team on Facebook for the slightest hint of what they might be thinking. Hadley was tired of TV—her dad would have been proud—and followed me from room to room as I switched off the sets. Finally, she spoke up.

"Mama, what's wrong? Why are you crying?"

She caught me off guard. This was definitely too much reality for my five-year-old.

"Um. Oh. Mommy is a little sad, honey."

"Why are you so sad, Mommy?"

"Well, babe, some people were running in a race, and they . . . they fell down and got hurt."

She was quiet for a minute.

"Did *all* the runners in the race fall down?"

I didn't know at first where she was going with that.

"No! Lots of the runners were just fine," I said.

That was enough for her. As she skipped out of the room, she called, "Well, then don't worry about the ones that fell down, Mommy! Everyone will help them up! That's what you guys do!"

Apparently, Hadley had been paying a whole lot of attention to my team stories—and she said the exact words I needed to hear. My runners weren't in Boston that day. My runners had not fallen down. But if they had been there, my team would have stopped without a moment's hesitation to help any one of the Boston Marathon victims. That really was what Team CMMD was about: the inherent goodness of the human spirit.

We may not have been there at the time of the bombings to lift up our fellow runners, but we would carry them on our backs and in our hearts on May 5. The event that had seemed to threaten our team's participation was the very same one that made our participation mandatory. And all it took for me to see it were the innocent words of an observant five-year-old.

The mass e-mail I typed was simple and short. I was honest about my own hesitations. I gave all of my forty-seven runners a free pass. I told them that I would understand if any one of them was reluctant to run, given the events of earlier that day. In closing, I spoke as the team captain: "Team CMMD will cross that finish line on May 5, 2013, even if that team has just two feet—mine."

I hovered my cursor for just a second over the SEND button and then clicked it with a flourish. I was relieved to have written the message, but then, once again, I was nervous. A bigger challenge loomed. I had to tell Chris and the kids that I would be running Broad Street as planned.

It is not often that Chris states his opinion with such conviction as to discourage any debate. I knew the moment he walked in that he knew all about Boston. His quiet smile was just the tiniest bit restrained. His normal hello hug lingered a split second longer than usual. I could see that he was sickened and saddened all at once. Chris let me go and scooped Hadley up, spinning her around while she told him about how "Mama was sad because some people fell down." His arms were wrapped tightly around her little body, and her face was buried against his neck. He didn't want to put her down, so instead he walked over to me and put his forehead against mine. "I love you," he whispered.

Hours later, when Hadley was finally asleep, I got up the courage to tell him my plan. He listened carefully as I recounted the battles my team had won, the personal accomplishments of my runners, and my conviction that we could not "let those bastards win!"

"Chris. I'm going to run—still."

He was quiet for a second, then said, "You are, huh?"

I braced myself. If there was anything he was a bulldog about, it was protecting me and the kids. I probably should have talked to him before I'd sent that e-mail to the team. . . . This decision could have serious consequences for our family.

"Am I missing something? When were you *not* going to run?"

"Well, yeah . . . today . . . after the bombings in Boston."

"You not running is not, and never was, an option. I know that, and you know that. Now you have to tell your team that."

After our nearly twenty years together, I had gotten pretty good at predicting how Chris would react to certain situations.

This was not the response I had expected. Chris was almost neurotic about our safety. When our children were babies, he would tiptoe in and lean his ear over their cribs to make sure they were breathing. As they got older, he would chase them down the street to remind them to put their helmets on. So for him not to forbid my participation in this road race was shocking.

Before I could tell him about my e-mail, my phone rang. It was TK, my nurse.

His voice cracked, and he cleared his throat. "Yo, boss lady. I'm in. See you tomorrow."

While I was on the phone with TK, I got a text message from another teammate.

"Oh. Hell. No. Those bastards aren't stopping me *or* us!"

The texts, e-mails, and voice messages trickled in all night. I was more and more uplifted and emboldened with each one. Before I went to bed, I had heard by phone, text, Facebook message, or e-mail from each and every runner on my team, and not one—not a single one—was opting out.

My runners were more than committed. They were determined. And now they were angry. Our donors kept donating and our supporters kept cheering. We heard from cancer widows who emptied closets and parents who had just bought tiny white caskets. "Run for my Mom . . . my Gabby . . . my daddy." With every donation and Facebook post of encouragement, we strengthened our resolve. Then, just three days after the Boston bombings, we got the ultimate plea in a Facebook post. It was from a cancer patient, but not just any patient. It was from Debi McLaughlin, one of the main reasons I had created my team in the first place.

On April 18 she wrote about the war that choroidal cancer—

a malignant melanoma of the eye—was waging against her body. She had tumors in her liver that had not responded to multiple procedures aimed at cutting off their blood supply. She explained that she was about to go in for yet another. She told us of her five small children and the husband she adored. She told us that she planned on being at the Broad Street Run finish line to hug us all.

My team rallied around Debi, promising to run their hearts out for her and her soon-to-be-motherless children. We hit the trails harder and faster than ever. We posted pleas on Facebook and sent mass e-mails again and again. Debi was quietly telling us that she understood it was too late for our efforts to do her any good, but it didn't have to be that way for another young family torn apart by cancer.

Less than two weeks before the race, we had raised $47,000. One day, Sam's baseball coach sent a check for $500. That was followed hours later by another $500 from an anonymous donor with the simple message "Thank you. Thank you. Thank you." The $50,000 mark was within our reach.

On April 23, 2013, with twelve days to go, our total stood at $49,653. At 10:00 that night, I asked my team to make another push . . . and I followed my plea with a promise. I would personally match every dollar raised before midnight.

As they had over and over again, my team came through. In two hours, we reached the $50,000 mark and the Meyer family was on the hook for $1,000. By April 25, 2013, we had raised more than twenty-five times my original goal, but I was tired. More than feeling just the muscle fatigue that came with training for a ten-mile race, I was mentally exhausted. Debi and Rosella were both failing their last-resort treatments. The embolizations that Debi had written us about had annihilated her liver function. Technically, it wasn't her metastatic melanoma that was killing her; it was her failing liver. That was one of the most brutal facts about cancer: often the treatment killed the patient before the cancer did. Rosella's breast cancer had recurred for the third time in as many years. This time, it was in the fluid around her lungs. Despite weekly procedures to drain it, that cancerous fluid was like a merciless tide—determined to drown her. And Joe Dunn's CEA level—the blood marker that indicated the presence of colon cancer cells—was on the rise. It was after the third exponential jump in that number that he decided to plan his own funeral.

Meanwhile, my aunt was scheduled for a procedure to reverse her colostomy. I knew how much she hated that bag she wore, but before it could be removed, doctors had to be sure she was cancer free. First, she would have a total-body CT scan and then a colonoscopy. They would do the colonoscopy only if the scans were clear. If she had tumors in her lungs or her liver, there would be no point in doing the scope; she would need more chemo. And she knew all about the lethality more chemo would have on her already-spent immune system. I was terrified that if her scans showed a recurrence, she would opt out of chemo and sign up to die when her cancer decided it was time.

Besides their ruthless cancers, Joe, Debi, Rosella, and my aunt had one other thing in common: me. And despite my unquestionable love for each of them, the wall of plaques in my office, and the tens of thousands of dollars my team had raised, in their stories, I was making absolutely zero difference. When it came down to it, in April 2013, I was many things—a devoted wife, an adoring mother, even an award-winning chef—but the one thing I aspired most to be, I was failing at.

I was anything but a good doctor.

It was this thought that played over and over in my mind on the short drive home just a few days before Broad Street. That sunny afternoon, I was so consumed by it, in fact, that I looked up and realized I was already making the turn onto my street and had no idea how I had gotten there.

As I stopped at the end of the driveway to pick up the mail, Hadley came bursting outside. Her skintight, pink leopard-print jeans were tucked into lighter-pink, faux-leather cowboy boots. It did not bother her in the least that the denim jacket she was crammed into had been a gift for her first birthday and hadn't fit her in three years, or that the boots were part of last Halloween's costume.

Hadley bounced around me as I sifted through catalogs, bills, and coupons. The carefully penned note was addressed to Dr. Christine Meyer. It was rare for me to get mail addressed to me professionally at home, and rarer yet for it to be handwritten. I tore open the envelope and stopped in the middle of the driveway, paralyzed by the first sentence.

Hi Christine,

This is Grace, your patient from US Air flight 964 on Easter Sunday. I just wanted to drop you a line to thank you again and let you know what happened to me after the flight.

From there, Grace Yatsko went on to describe the events that had taken place starting the moment she had deplaned on a stretcher a month before. The ambulance had taken her right to Methodist, a small community hospital near the airport. There, Grace was deemed too ill for that hospital's resources and was subsequently transported to Jefferson, the world-class teaching hospital where I had trained, and where Grace learned that she had suffered a heart attack affecting the right side of her heart.

It all came together in my mind. Coincidentally, the same cardiology team from Jefferson that had taken over Grace's care had trained me nearly twenty years before.

It had been on grueling 6:00 A.M. rounds with Michael Savage, MD, that I'd learned the very lesson that may have helped save Grace's life. In a heart attack affecting the *left* side of the heart, administering IV fluids can be lethal—the patient's weakened heart will not be able to pump excess fluid, and they will suffer from pulmonary edema, essentially drowning.

That morning, Dr. Savage chose me as the recipient of the question "Dr. Meyer, Mr. Liacouras is in respiratory distress. Can you tell us why?"

"Um. He had a heart attack.... He's not mobilizing fluids.... He has pulmonary edema." I stammered, but I knew I was right.

"You are half right," Dr. Savage said. "The piece you are missing, Doctor, is that *you* tried to drown him last night." He was not smiling. "Mr. Liacouras had a left-sided heart attack. His blood pressure dropped because of the morphine he was getting for pain. You ordered a wide-open bag of normal saline. His heart couldn't handle it, and he nearly died. Thankfully, your chief caught the mistake and gave the patient a diuretic."

My chief resident looked smug. I was going to pay for that mistake later.

Suddenly, Dr. Savage's face softened and he continued, "If you take away one lesson from my rotation, let it be this one: In a *right*-sided heart attack, fluids will save a life. In a left, they will cost one. You have only a short window to decide, so choose carefully."

I recalled that horrible morning in the hospital, and then my performance on flight 964 weeks before. My decision to give Grace fluids was largely reflexive. Unlike in normal medical situations, I had no data—no ECG, no blood tests, no oxygen meter. All I had was one of the few sentences Grace had been able to share with us that day: "I got nauseous and fainted." Nausea was a classic symptom of *right*-sided heart attack.

Grace concluded her letter with:

> *I truly believe that angels do exist. I make the enclosed angel cards and carry them when I fly and give them out to all the pilots, copilots, and flight attendants. Not only do I hand them out, but I say the prayer over and over while flying. On flight 964, God not only had the angels fly beneath the wings of the plane but also placed three in the plane: you, Jackie, and Paul [the flight attendant who assisted us on the plane]. If it were not for the three of you, chances are, I would not be here today.*
>
> *I know my situation is nothing compared with the devastation that happened to those poor people in Boston this past week. I have and will keep them in my daily prayers, along with you, Jackie, and Paul.*

I will be eternally indebted to you. Thank you again,
and God bless you.

Sincerely,
Grace Yatsko

And just like that, my rambling thoughts of futility and my uselessness to Debi, Rosella, Joe, and Tant gave way to just one: *I* am *a good doctor.*

The week after I received Grace Yatsko's letter, I heard from Tant. Her scans and scope were clear. She would be having her colostomy reversed in the next few days. When I asked what I could do for her, Tant responded the way she always did. "Don't worry about me. I'm fine." This time, in my heart, I believed her.

Chapter 12: THE LONGEST MILE

The miracle isn't that I finished.

The miracle is that I had the courage to start.

—John Bingham

R unning a ten-mile race is a lot like being pregnant. For the first third of the race, you wonder why you decided to do this. You feel nauseous, weak, and terrified—you may even vomit. And, at least once or twice in those first three miles, you feel certain that you will die before the godforsaken thing is done.

Somewhere around the third or fourth mile, your mood shifts. You get into a groove. You look up instead of down. Your shoulders spread and your mind clears. You feel light, fit, and beautiful. Certainly, those around you wonder whether you are an Olympic athlete. You vow to run every ten-miler in town for an entire year. You add a half marathon to your list of life goals.

Then, as you come to the seventh mile, the magic stops. Your legs feel like anvils. You must have gained a hundred pounds just since you started this leg. Your hands and feet are puffy, your bra straps are too tight, and for the life of you, you cannot get the urge to pee out of your mind. You start to loathe everyone around you—especially the chipper ones. To the spry young man who just blew past you and smiled, you say, "Screw you!"—out loud. You are certain this race is the worst decision you've ever made. If you survive, your life will never be the same. But you are trapped now. You cannot go back. Your only choice is to go forward, to see it to the end. You may pull over and sit on the ground and cry for a second, but then you go on.

Finally, you are in that ninth mile. You have come so far. *What's another mile?* you say to yourself. Well, another mile is like being two weeks overdue in August, in Alabama—just about unbearable.

The difference between finishing a ten-mile race and giving birth is simply in the reward. At the end of the race, you will have put all of your hopes and dreams into a cheap medal and a free banana—neither of which will cure cancer or win you a Pulitzer.

* * *

To most of us on Team CMMD, race day arrived with little pomp and ceremony. Running coaches love to say that after months of training, the actual race is just a "victory lap." The key word there is "lap." No lap is ten miles. And after all that we had done and been through, almost all of us would have gladly skipped a victory lap and gone straight to the post-race margaritas.

But of course we were going to run.

We had stayed up most of the night before, writing the

names of our loved ones in Sharpie on silk ribbons, which we pinned to the backs of our shirts. Red ribbons honored cancer survivors and fighters; white ones honored those who had fallen. Some had so many, so carefully placed, that they formed capes that flowed behind their wearers like Superman's. One girl had a solitary ribbon pinned to her back, and the three letters scrawled on it broke my heart: "Dad."

I wrote out my ribbons slowly and carefully, taking time to think about every name as I carefully spelled it out. I was thankful that they were mostly red but knew in my soul that had the race happened just a bit later, at least three of my red ribbons—the ones for Joe, Debi, and Rosella—would have been white.

I saved Tant's ribbon for last. She had finished her chemo, she had clear scans, she had had her colostomy reversed, and she was about to do what she had missed most in her months of treatment: she was going back to work. As I pinned her red ribbon to the carefully chosen center spot, I stared at her real name: Venis Fanous, MD. Yes, her patients needed her, but that wasn't all—*I* needed her. I grabbed another red ribbon and carefully penned "Tant" on it.

* * *

Our plan for race day was well laid and communicated. Team CMMD would gather at my office, where we would board a school bus to the Broad Street start line, in the Olney section of Philadelphia.

The day before, I had picked up a box full of all forty-seven of my runners' race-day packets. After Boston, the Philadelphia

Parks Commission had issued a statement about enhanced security at the Broad Street Run. Only runners with bibs would be allowed anywhere near the secure race areas. Besides providing access to the race, the bibs were fitted with individual computerized chips that would track our time and pace. Without those bibs, we would not be able to run, and all of our training would have been for nothing.

I left the box in my trunk and locked the car. On race-day morning, I breathed a sigh of relief as I pulled out the familiar parcel, envelopes overflowing. I had half expected the box to disappear. All night, I had tossed fitfully, worrying that none of my runners would run because I had failed to get them their bibs.

The empty school bus arrived right on time for our 5:45 A.M. departure. I stood in the middle of my packed waiting room with the large cardboard box at my feet and cleared my throat. "Listen up, guys!" The room quieted.

"I am going to call out your names, and you'll come up, grab your packet, and head out to the bus."

I reached down and pulled out the first envelope. Jeffrey Adams was not a name I recognized. No one came forward. Neither did Angela Mastroly, George Hoffman, or Erica Hoover. I picked up envelope after envelope, only to throw them all on the ground. Panic filled me. These were not our bibs. This was not our box. *Oh my God.*

Now the room was really quiet. Arlen came over. "What's up?" he whispered. He sounded the way he had when he'd told me about the missing cilantro.

"I-I don't have our bibs. This isn't our box. . . ." Now my voice was shaking and I was certain I was about to faint.

"Stay calm," Arlen cooed, though he knew as well as I did that we had no chance of getting those bibs now. We were barely going to make it to the start line in time as it was. There was no race-day-pickup option for this run. Unlike other races, where you could pay a bit extra to get your bib the morning of the race, because of Broad Street's sheer number of runners (forty-one thousand) and the enhanced security at the start and finish lines, its organizers insisted that all bibs be picked up no later than the day before the run.

I put my face in my hands. I felt frozen in place. I don't remember who it was, but someone suddenly started dumping the contents of the box all over the floor, and then I heard Arlen's voice call out a name.

"Wendy Ford?" Wendy bounded over and grabbed her envelope with a grin. I looked up, and Wendy winked at me. I remembered how, the day of the food fight, she had dropped everything to help me peel ten pounds of shallots. Wendy Ford was and would always be the heart and soul of this team.

Once the box had been emptied, it became clear that someone had tossed a bunch of random bibs on *top*. Our team's bibs—all forty-seven of them—were underneath the random ones.

Although I felt as though an hour had passed during the bib debacle, in reality we were only a few minutes behind schedule. I started to clean up the carnage of discarded bibs on the floor, when I came across one for Patty Dungan. Patty was actually the fifth runner to join our team; she had signed on right after TK, Clare-E, Joan, and me. But she had not yet appeared today to claim her bib or her seat on the bus.

I looked at my watch. It was 6:00 A.M. We were fifteen minutes late, and Patty was nowhere to be found. The bus was idling and full, except for two seats: mine and Patty's. As I climbed the steps to board, the driver gave me an exasperated look, as if to say, *Look, lady, you busted my balls about getting outta here on time, and now we're waiting on you. You got some nerve.*

I decided to try my sweet, mild-mannered persona for this one. "Um, hi. What was your name, again? Oh. Well, Joe, I'm Christine." I put my hand out. Joe took it with the stunned but pleasantly surprised look of someone being handed a wad of cash.

"We are short one runner. Can we wait a minute or two?" The team was busy laughing and carrying on. TK had torn the sleeves of his running T-shirt and was busy kissing each of his biceps in an unabashed display of manliness. For post-run "hydration," some runners had decided to bring buckets of premixed margaritas, which they promptly began filling with tequila.

It took a second for me to get the team's attention. "Hey! We're missing Patty Dungan. Has anyone heard from her?"

As everyone dug around for their phone, I was reminded to check mine. I had been so busy with the bibs that I'd missed a text from Patty. Four words and a sad-face emoji: "Overslept. Go without me." She had sent it seven minutes before.

I fired off, "No way! *Hurry!* We won't leave without you."

I had no sooner hit SEND than Patty's red Jeep came careening into the parking lot and screeched to a stop, straddling two parking spots—both handicapped spaces.

The cheers for Patty, who scrambled onto the bus with the finesse of an aging elephant, were quickly replaced by shrieks of laughter. Patty was juggling her keys, phone, and . . . sneakers. In her rush to make the bus, she had raced out of the house barefoot. Ironically, despite her rocky start, Patty would finish

Broad Street with one of the best times of anyone on the team. She was a rocket!

With Patty aboard, bibs distributed, energy shots drunk, and tequila mixed, I collapsed in the front seat and closed my eyes, believing I did not have a ten-mile run in me—not after the morning, the week, and the year I'd had.

It was a cloudy and chilly morning, but the forecast called for temperatures near seventy and sunny skies later in the day. One of the greatest traditions of Philly distance runs was the "sweats shed." Since it was often much cooler at the start of a race and runners tended to heat up once they got moving, all participants were invited to wear layers and discard them along the race route as they warmed up. Later, massive cleaning crews would ride the course, collecting all the warm clothes, which they would then launder and donate to homeless shelters.

So that morning, all forty-seven of us, along with tens of thousands of other runners, donned our old college sweats, and clothes we simply *never* needed to see our husbands wear again.

Joe, the reluctant Krapf's coach driver, had agreed to get us as close to the start line of the Broad Street Run as possible and then turn around and park somewhere near the finish line, where we would all board the bus back home. From the bus, our first stop was the porta-potties: a notorious aspect of the Philadelphia Broad Street Run. The city boasted that eight hundred portable toilets would be available before, during, and after the race. We all split up in search of the shortest lines. After bouncing around in the cold and urgently needing to pee, I finally got my turn. The guy coming out of the stall gave me an apologetic look, like he had done some serious business in that john. I sucked in a deep breath and went in.

I am a physician and a mother. I have had people throw up, bleed, and pee directly on parts of my person. Yet nothing— *nothing*—prepared me for the utter filth in that portable stall, where I learned quickly about "runner's diarrhea"—what runners call the urgent, almost uncontrollable need to defecate during a run. However, I always thought it was something that happened while you were actually *running*—not an event that took place an hour before the race even started.

As much as I tried to avert my gaze, my eyes fell first on the abyss beneath the wet seat. There was no longer any identifiable blue water, only mountains of excrement still steaming in the chilly air. There was no way I was going to let my bare skin make contact with the toilet seat, so I opted for an air squat, pulling the collar of my bleach-stained Champion sweatshirt over my mouth and nose while I hovered precariously.

I looked up at the inside of the door and was struck by the idiocy of the sign on it: THIS UNIT IS MEANT TO SERVICE TEN PEO-PLE DURING A NORMAL FORTY-HOUR WORK WEEK. Clearly, it was not meant to service fifty runners with irritable bowel syndrome.

The imagery only worsened from there. To my right, the tiny built-in urinal was bone dry and empty, save for the smallest blue urinal cake. It was so small and sad, it could actually have been a lone Smarty candy. Of course the urinal was pristine—no one was peeing; they were all unloading hundreds of pounds of crap. The sick gray plastic wall to my left held an empty toilet paper roll—I guessed I would need to shake and dry. Then there was the wall unit of hand sanitizer. In the late 1990s, studies showed that in hospitals, doctors and nurses were so bad at washing their hands with soap and water that they failed to remove 90 percent of the bacteria on them. We were spreading deadly infections to our hospitalized patients because of ineffective hand washing. Enter the alcohol-based hand-sanitizer movement. Rates of hospital-acquired infections plummeted. But, alas, this particular hand-sanitizer unit would do very little to stem the tide of sickness, as it was itself covered in excrement.

I pulled up my running skirt and kicked open the door, stumbling out like a smoke-inhalation victim leaving a burning building. I caught the eye of the girl behind me and said, "Um, it's really gross in there . . . and there's no toilet paper." She gave me a sympathetic look, but I could tell she didn't exactly believe me. All I could do was run away in search of my teammates and hope never, ever to lay eyes on her again.

The sheer number of Broad Street runners made it impossible for everyone to start at the same time. Corral assignments divided runners into groups according to their anticipated finish time. Faster runners were positioned in corrals nearest the start line, and slower runners brought up the rear. The vast majority of our runners were positioned in the farthest-back corrals, so most of us hadn't even started the run by the time the faster runners were crossing the finish line. I made my way past the elite runners—the ones who would finish the ten-mile race in less than an hour—and kept strolling back from the start line for about ten minutes, until I found the gray corral, designating the second-slowest group. Behind me was the pink corral. I was annoyed that the color pink identified the slowest group; I knew for a fact that there were several women on my team who could outrun any dude.

As I squeezed next to an elderly woman, I scanned the crowd

for another shocking-green Team CMMD shirt. I thought I saw a few, but they were way behind me, I would never get to them in time, as the corrals were gradually moving toward the start line. The race was about to start, and despite having created, encouraged, supported, and coordinated the winningest fund-raising team in the history of that race, I found myself about to run all alone.

I checked my phone, hoping to text a teammate to meet me. Although I had excellent cell reception, I could not successfully transmit a text or make a call. I looked around. Hundreds of people were staring at their phones, then looking up at the sky in puzzlement. The sheer volume of people congregated in that small area was overwhelming cell towers. Resigned to the fact that I would start alone, I put my wireless headphones in my ears and slid my phone into my skirt pocket. Then I did what all runners do in the moments before a race start: I bent down to tie my laces one last time. As I crouched, I looked ahead at all the hundreds of feet in front of me, and for a moment, my breath caught. In every direction, my ground-level view caught one image repeated: red socks. I glanced down at my own pair, recalling with sadness and fear the bombings at the Boston Marathon two weeks before.

The clean melody of OneRepublic's "I Lived" filled my ears. The song's message of living life to its fullest and never giving up drowned out the crowd and reminded me that I was running despite my own grief for Debi, Rosella, Joe, Tant, the runners of the Boston Marathon, and thousands of others. Despite those lowest of moments, I would persevere.

I thought of Martin Richard, the eight-year-old boy who was killed instantly while he waited for his dad at the Boston

Marathon finish line on April 15, 2013. He was just feet away from his twin sister and older brother. I thought of Adrianne Haslet-Davis, the young woman whose left foot was blown off the instant the first bomb went off. If she survived, she might never again do what she was passionate about—dance. I thought of Debi and Rosella and Joe, getting ready to take their final falls. I thought of their loves, wishes, fears, and pain. And when my feet were over the start line, I remembered my very first run—the five-miler that made a runner out of me.

My right foot stepped on the mat, the chip in my bib was activated, I felt electricity course through my body, from my toes to my scalp, and I began to cry. For the first couple of miles, I stumbled along, not really able to run efficiently while wiping my nose and eyes with the sleeve of my old sweatshirt. My team seemed to have vanished. Coincidentally, much as I had vowed to in the e-mail after Boston, it appeared that I would in fact be crossing the finish line alone. As sobering as that thought was, being without a teammate had its advantages. I found myself acutely aware of my surroundings. Despite having run that very same course before, I had not ever actually *seen* it. In that northern stretch, the crowd was made up almost entirely of minorities. Older women sat in wheelchairs. Church choirs gathered on steps to serenade us as we passed. One young man with an entrepreneurial spirit pushed a shopping cart full of unwrapped Philly soft pretzels and bottles of water. I laughed, wondering how hungry someone would have to be to eat one of those pretzels.

From the start line, Broad Street runs south through the grittiest parts of North Philadelphia, where fast-food joints share curb space with check-cashing stores. That day, the police and military presence was palpable. At every cross-street, two uniformed and armed officers stood guard. I found myself stopping for just a few moments to remove one earbud and shout, "Thank you!" to each man and woman in uniform along the way. They mostly smiled and nodded. Early on, just as I picked up my pace and before I had replaced my earbud, one called after me, "No, thank *you!*" I looked back to see the middle-aged officer motioning to my shirt full of ribbons. It was the spirit of all of these people—officers and citizens alike—that pushed me along in those early miles.

Temple University Hospital is a world-class teaching hospital planted in the middle of a war zone. That section of Philadelphia consistently has some of the worst crime statistics in the state and the country. But not that day. On the first Sunday of every May, the thousands of runners and spectators became great equalizers. The day of this run, Broad Street was just Broad Street—no matter what stretch or what neighborhood. Outside the hospital, dozens of patients sat in parked wheelchairs, thin hospital blankets wrapped around jutting shoulders. Needle-battered arms—some still hooked up to bags of fluids—were lifted with great effort to cheer runners on as they passed. Those wheelchairs reminded me of my good fortune: two working legs, my lack of cancer, my foot—spared instantaneous amputation by a psychopath's bomb. Alongside the patient spectators stood sleep-deprived resident physicians, white lab coats stained with coffee and bearing the telltale wrinkles of having been slept in. I ran passed those exhausted, unshaven faces and sent a telepathic message: *Hang in there. This will be over soon, and it will be worth it. You will be doctors. You will make a difference someday.*

I chose the water station near Temple to check my music

and take a breather. As I fumbled with my phone, I noticed my Twitter icon. I would tweet my way down Broad! I didn't care about my time, and I had no one near me to hurry me along. Just after Temple Hospital, the scrubs and dirty white coats gave way to maroon-colored football uniforms. For the next mile or two, I could feel the sting in my palms—a reminder of the high fives I accepted enthusiastically from the enormous young men who made up that team. I felt amazing, on top of the world, downright exhilarated. *That* would be my first tweet.

I didn't stop to think that tweeting while running, crying, and exhausted might make for some typing inaccuracies. Later, I would deeply regret that first, impromptu post. Hours after the race ended, an older patient of mine, who had been there to watch the run, approached me and said, "Hey there, Doc. Looks like you had one hell of a time up at Temple!"

Is he confused? Is he referring to my med school days? Should I correct him and tell him that I went to Hahnemann, not Temple?

Later, I looked over my tweets and in a moment of utter mortification understood what the old man was referring to. My first tweet of the race was meant to read: "I just high-fived the entire Temple football team at mile 4!"—only "high-fived" had been autocorrected to "had," and it now read: "I just *had* the entire Temple football team at mile 4!"

True to our team spirit, all sorts of commentary would flow from that tweet, including theories about why I enjoyed running in skirts and not-so-subtle implications about how I had *really* raised all that money. Later on, whenever I complained of being worn-out or tired, someone on the team was always sure to ask whether there had been a football team in my near past.

* * *

At City Hall, the check-cashing kiosks gave way to the high-rises of Philadelphia's financial district, and politicians and suburbanites, there to cheer on loved ones, replaced our elderly, sick, tired, and boisterous spectators. A little girl not older than five proudly held up a hand-drawn sign that read GO MOM! I thought of the cheering on flight 964 and the pride in my own kids' voices as they called, "Way to go, Mom!" and again tears sprang to my eyes. I wished they were there. I wished I could see Chris's warm smile or my Hadley bobbing up and down excitedly. But even before the Boston Marathon bombings, Chris had decided the Philadelphia Broad Street Run, with its forty-one thousand participants and tens of thousands of spectators, was no place for our children.

A few feet down the road, a young man in loose-fitting jeans, black-rimmed glasses, and flip-flops caught my eye. His meticulous stubble implied careful attention to detail, not dishevelment. I was so consumed by his appearance that I almost missed the sign he held up: IF BROAD STREET WERE EASY, IT WOULD BE YOUR MOTHER.

I was still laughing when I looked up to find myself passing the Academy of Music. Built in 1857, it remains the oldest still-running opera house in the United States. On a warm, sunny June afternoon in 1997, I had received my medical degree inside that grand auditorium. What took place that day was much more than a commencement; it included a formal "hooding" ceremony, traditional for advanced degrees and doctoral programs. Rather than handing students symbolic scrolls of parchment, faculty place a revered hood of thick velvet over the head of each graduate. Once the hood is in place and draped just so over the silk graduation robe, the doctorate is considered complete.

As I ran past the Academy, I recalled Hahnemann's beloved tradition. Family members with doctoral degrees were invited to be honorary faculty members and "hood" their loved ones. When I first invited Tant to hood me, she seemed hesitant and replied, "But I don't know how to do that!" Her protestations were thin and short-lived, however, and on graduation day she took her place on the stage alongside my anatomy, physiology, and histology professors. When my name was called, she stood up confidently and walked to the front of the stage with me. She then stood behind me in the full faculty regalia and gently placed the hallowed hood around my neck. I had to duck a little so that she wouldn't have to reach too far. I felt like the luckiest girl in the world: Chris was just ahead of me, and the doctor I had spent a lifetime learning from was bestowing my hard-earned reward upon me.

Most faculty advisors shook hands with their graduate. Not Tant. She planted a soft kiss on my cheek and whispered, "You did it, Cat, but this is not the end; it is just the beginning. One day, you will make a difference. It may be a big difference or it may be small, but I promise you, one day you *will* make a difference."

That thought filled my mind at the seventh mile as I neared Methodist Hospital—the very one Grace Yatsko, my accidental patient from flight 964, had been taken to from the airport. She had been transferred from Methodist to Jefferson, just a few miles up the road, for more intensive care. I remembered my days as the medical admitting resident in Jefferson's ER, where my number-one job was not to admit sick patients but to protect my fellow medical residents from admissions. Admissions meant more work on top of workloads that were already barely manageable. And the absolute worst admissions were the transfers from other, "lesser" hospitals, such as Methodist.

Back then, patients like Grace would have made our lives as medical residents hard. None of us had the insight to see that those patients were also teaching us lifelong lessons or that those "lesser" hospitals were where patients were truly saved. These smaller, less-lauded facilities were the ones that stabilized the sickest patients enough for the "hotshots" at places like Jefferson to take over and ultimately take credit for those patients' favorable outcomes.

Shortly after passing Methodist, I hit the proverbial wall. I was exhausted. I ate my energy goo and drank my Gatorade. I changed my music and dumped a cup of water, enthusiastically shoved at me by a young volunteer, on my head. Nothing was working; I could not will my legs to move.

Then I saw him.

Coming up on my right was a man about my age. He seemed to be in pain. Not only was he obviously hurting, but he was also hobbling. It took me a minute to figure out why. He was an amputee and was running on a prosthetic limb.

I loathed myself at that moment. *Jesus Christ, this guy has one goddamn leg and he's still running. . . . I. Have. Got. To. Move. My. Ass.*

With a dramatic flair, I crushed my empty cup in one hand and slammed it onto the ground, where it landed with the thousands of other trampled Solo cups. As I pulled up next to the one-legged runner, I put my hand on his shoulder and smiled. "You got this!" I called.

He smiled back in quiet thanks, and then his face changed. We were only about two miles from the finish line. My plan became to "hold back" and finish the run side by side with him, even if it meant sacrificing a few minutes on my personal time. My resolve to help a struggling fellow runner was invigorating; after all, Hadley had reminded me, *that* was what we did on this team.

My joy didn't last long, though—in a blink, my new running mate found his groove, one without me in it. He took off ahead of me and within seconds was completely out of my range of vision. An amputee on a prosthetic leg had just smoked me. And boy, did it feel good.

Just before the ninth mile, the crowd came alive. Perfect strangers cheered loudly. They caught my eye and screamed at me to keep going. They called, "You are *so close!*" and, "One. More. Mile!" and, "Go, girl!"

I was certain each and every one of them was speaking right to me and only me.

Then someone was.

When I first heard it, I thought my fatigue and dehydration were causing me to hallucinate, but then I heard it again: a soft, straining voice.

"Dr. Meyer . . . Dr. Meyer . . . *Christine!*"

Sitting in a wheelchair on the opposite side of the wide stretch of road, wrapped in a shawl, squinting her one good eye against the glare of the sun, was Debi McLaughlin. Just as she had that day in my waiting room—the last time I had seen her—she was calling my name again. She had done as she had promised and was there at the finish to cheer us—to cheer me—on.

I was too far over to the left of the path, and there were too many runners between us; I wouldn't be able to get to her. So, as sheer momentum propelled my body forward, I jumped up and down and waved my arms, praying that Debi would see me and know that I had seen her.

My dear, dying patient, nearing her own finish line, had made the trek to cheer me to mine. I wanted to curl up next to her and squeeze the cancer out of her. I wanted to make her better. I wanted her not to die.

Finishing the Broad Street Run was one of the hardest things I have ever had to do. After I passed Debi, I was done. I had expended every last bit of my emotional energy. I didn't care about the race, the money, or the team, but Debi had come out to see me finish, so I had to finish—for her.

I ran that last mile of Broad Street one step at a time. With every strike of my throbbing feet, I thought of Debi, Joe, Rosella, Tant, Grace, the Boston victims, and my team. Names, faces, and stories flashed through my mind as though it were *my* life that was ending. Memories, images, my aunt's words, Rosella's cross, Debi's smile—all flooded me, each one reigniting a spark I thought I had lost four miles, six months, and a lifetime ago, and I picked up speed, feeling at times as if my feet were barely grazing the pavement.

As the Navy Yard gates entered my view and the crowd grew even louder and thicker, I came to a conclusion that altered the course of my life from that moment forward. This longest mile wasn't the end of my journey; it was the beginning.

Epilogue

Our deepest fear is not that we are inadequate.

Our deepest fear is that we are powerful beyond measure.

It is our light, not our darkness, that most frightens us.

—Marianne Williamson

The Team

I felt as though I glided in slow motion over the finish line that day. Enthusiastic faces shouted inaudible words. I remember vivid yet inconsequential details about some of those people: the way saliva sprayed in an arc as one man turned his head to call out to me; the immaculately manicured nails of a lady holding up a sign; the dripping lollipop in a little girl's hands as she sat perched on her dad's shoulders. In my mind, I would replay these snapshots again and again over the coming months and years.

On that day, May 5, 2013, after a brief celebration at the finish-line tents, we made the trek to our school bus. Unfortunately, we had underestimated the sheer number of identical yellow buses that many of the forty-one thousand other runners would use for their own transportation. Later, we figured that our "walk" to the bus added at least three miles to the ten we had just run—in other words, we'd completed a half marathon.

When we finally identified our idling bus, our sweaty bodies huddled together on board. While it was not hot, the sheer stench of our team mandated that every window be open for the ninety-minute ride home. I leaned my head back and closed my eyes, thinking back on the long road to the ten-mile race we had all just finished: four runners to forty-seven; Tant's life-threatening diagnosis to her triumphant recovery; deep desperation to eternal hope.

A few hours later, over one hundred people would gather at my house for a celebratory postrace picnic that almost didn't happen. I had chosen the week right after the food fight to "ask" Chris if it would be all right to host this gathering at our home. It wasn't really an ask, though, because I would not take no for an answer—although no was precisely what he said.

"Cat, I love you and am proud of you and all you have accomplished, but I need our home and family back for a while. I do not want to spend another Sunday with my house full of strangers."

At the time, we came to a compromise: I would host the party as long as he didn't have to be there. So the planning commenced, invites were sent, and RSVPs were counted. All in all, we were expecting 112 guests. Chris repeatedly stood his ground. "Good luck, sounds fun . . . but remember, I won't be there." Then it was the night before the race and the party, and as he watched me fill coolers with ice and beer, I looked up and began to cry. "I can't believe you're going to miss this after everything that's happened. How could you *not* be here?"

Chris shook his head and walked away. I knew I was reneging on my promise, but I wanted him by my side.

Because of the bus-finding fiasco, we got out of Philly later than we had anticipated and arrived at my house to find several of our friends and family members, along with Brad, the barbecue-pit master we had hired for the occasion, already waiting for us. By early afternoon, the clouds had cleared and the sky was a crystal blue. I sucked in my breath as I walked into my backyard, which my neighbor and dear friend Danielle had magically transformed. Dozens of tables set with cloths in our team colors dotted the long, narrow space. Two buffet tables were loaded with enough hearty fare to make even this group of exhausted and starving runners happy.

I saw his signature baseball cap before I saw him. Chris was sitting with Tom and Amy O'Grady. He leaned back in his chair and took a long swig from his cold bottle of beer. He was laughing and relaxed. He was here.

Despite the massive amounts of lactic acid in my legs, I galloped down the deck steps to where he sat and threw my arms around his neck. Chris stood up and lifted me off the ground and spun me around. "How did you do?" he asked.

It didn't matter. The race. The time. The team. The money. At that moment, the only important thing was that he was here. Again, I was crying.

It so happened that the 2013 Broad Street Run took place on May 5: Cinco de Mayo. An assortment of frozen margaritas would naturally complement the feast of ribs, baked beans, and coleslaw we had planned. Later, I would blame three of those cocktails for my tear-filled speech—one that would set the course for Team CMMD and inconceivable accomplishments.

Standing on my backyard patio, I turned toward the bright sun and let the breeze smooth my hair off my face. The lead singer of the band handed me a microphone, which I took eagerly. Chris smiled at me and winked. Words tumbled out of my mouth as if pulled by an outside force. I thanked the team and their families. I reminded everyone that our forty-seven runners had raised over $65,000, and then I said, "And I don't know about you, but I kind of feel like we're just getting started . . . Broad Street 2014!

"Ten miles.

"One hundred runners.

"One hundred thousand dollars.

"Yes. We. Can!"

A tray of used plastic dishes and forks crashed way up in the kitchen, breaking the momentary silence my announcement had induced. The crowd then let out a collective groan, followed by rousing applause. I had just announced, out loud, to over a hundred people, that the following year my goal would be to recruit one hundred runners and to raise $100,000.

Among those celebrating with us was Jamie Stanek, a self-proclaimed *non*-runner. He and his wife, Shannon, a local veterinarian, had been die-hard supporters of our team, but neither of them ran. Well, something in Jamie was stirred that day. Not only did he join the 2014 team (vowing only to *walk*, never run), but he did in fact start running. Jamie completed Broad Street in 2014 and again in 2015. And then this "nonrunner" went on to finish several half marathons. He has became a voice of leadership, humor, and inspiration for our team.

For the weeks following the 2013 Broad Street Run's post-race party, I continued to blame exhaustion, excitement, and margaritas for my ill-conceived delusions of grandeur, but it was too late. "It" was out there. No American Cancer Society DetermiNation running team had ever even come close to achieving the challenge I had posed to my team: to double our numbers and raise $100,000 in *one* Broad Street Run season.

Over the summer and fall, the original Team CMMD began recruiting friends and family for our 2014 effort. By Broad Street Run race day, the following May 4, we had 154 registered runners. That 2014 team crossed the Broad Street finish line having raised $174,000.

Despite having trained hard for that run, I almost didn't make it to the finish line myself. As I approached the mile-nine marker, I caught sight of a family gathered by the side of the road, holding signs that read GO CMMD! Immediately, I recognized the tall, clean-shaven man as Bob McLaughlin, Debi's widower. I quickly made my way over to where he, Debi's sister, brother, parents, and five kids stood and hugged them one by one. When I came face-to-face with Debi's mom and looked into her tired, sad eyes, I thought of my own mother and daughters and began to cry. Neither of us uttered one word, but she held me tight as deep sobs racked both of our bodies. I felt as if many minutes had passed before she gently and silently pushed me back onto the racecourse. Of the thousands of miles I had logged over the years, the last mile of the 2014 Broad Street Run was the hardest I have ever run.

One year later, our team of 154 had become 1,200. The original $67,000 we raised for the ACS that first year was simply the seed for the nearly $500,000 we raised over the subsequent two years. Yet, despite all the money we've contributed to fighting cancer, our biggest team accomplishment has actually been our *team*.

Hundreds of people who never dreamed they could even walk a mile trained and ran ten. Many cancer fighters joined our ranks and ran despite surgery, radiation, and chemo. Earl Dering Jr., the skin cancer survivor who showed up at our first-ever group run, kept on running. Not only did Earl become a really fast runner, he even completed the Marine Corps marathon. His story—nonrunner to marathoner, all while he had multiple surgeries for an aggressive squamous cell cancer on his face—inspired hundreds of people to lace up their shoes. In fact, at the time of this book's publication, the American Cancer Society's Team DetermiNation has just recruited Earl to be a running mentor—and his story is only one of many just like it.

On a Thursday in June 2015, Amy, a cancer fighter in the middle of her chemotherapy, announced on Facebook that she would join us for a few "slow" ones the next morning at 5 am. The team, awed by her strength, came out in droves. Over fifty-five people ran that early morning—not just *for* Amy but *because* of Amy.

After our second Broad Street Run, we began holding monthly dedication runs. On those Sundays, we honor one or two cancer warriors or angels. After a brief introduction about who we are running for, runners and walkers take off down the trail. Some run fast, some slowly. Some log just a mile, and some ten or more. Yet all of us run with one thing in common and in our hearts and minds: those cancer warriors and angels.

One cold February night, I wrote a post on Facebook encouraging my team to come out the next morning. The forecast called for bitter temperatures. I reminded everyone to wear gloves and face masks and to bring headlamps. "Yes, running in the dark in ten degrees is hard . . . but you all know what's harder, right?" The unspoken answer—*cancer is harder*—became a battle cry for our team. Seventy-eight people showed up the next, frigid morning, and our pictures of frozen eyelashes and icicles in sweaty hairlines became a Facebook sensation.

The Food Fight

It turns out our first food fight would be dwarfed by the next two. Food Fight 2 netted over $30,000, and Food Fight 3 raised over $67,000. As of this writing, plans are under way for Food Fight 4 to feature two world-renowned celebrity chefs going head-to-head against my team of amateurs. What started out as a friendly kitchen competition has become the most highly anticipated charity event in our community.

The Patients

Debi and Rosella both lost their battles with cancer within weeks of Broad Street 2013 and just days apart. In January 2014, Joe Dunn died. In less than one year, I lost all three of the patients who inspired me to tell this story, but I am fortunate to be in contact with all of their families, who remain staunch supporters of Team CMMD and our mission.

At the time of this book's publication, Karen Baker, our auction chair and liposarcoma sufferer, has endured over half a dozen surgeries, including a below-the-hip amputation. She continues to fight her cancer and will remain on chemotherapy for the foreseeable future. In May 2015, Team CMMD Foundation created the Karen Baker Scholarship, a $20,000 scholarship to be presented annually to a graduating senior whom cancer has impacted. The first Karen Baker Scholarship was awarded to Megan Brideau, who lost her father to kidney cancer. This young woman moved us to tears as we read her application essay.

"If I want to remember all of the amazing things about him, I have to be amazing. . . . If I ever become a fraction of what my dad was, I can be happy in my life." Many of us carry those words with us, striving to be just a bit of what our heroes were.

The Foundation

Early in 2015, Team CMMD Foundation officially became a publicly recognized 501(c)(3) charity. Our expanded mission is to support local cancer families while continuing to raise money for large, nongovernmental funders of cancer research, like the American Cancer Society.

Key players from that first year make up Team CMMD Foundation's leadership. Kristy Harper, my friend who started a massive fund-raising rally with her $2,000 donation, is now our vice chair. Rebekah Ulmer, the food fight photographer who suffered a massive stroke less than one year after the event, not only beat the odds—she was given just a 5 percent chance of survival—but now serves as our communications director.

In the early fall of 2014, we unveiled the first Team CMMD in Training program. Over sixty kids between the ages of seven and twelve completed a nine-week 5K training program. On November 15, 2014, they, along with nearly eight hundred other individuals, completed the first annual Team CMMD 5K, called This Run's Personal.

As I write this epilogue, Team CMMD Foundation has given tens of thousands of dollars to local families reeling from the effects of cancer.

Our running team has also expanded to include a cycling arm. In June 2015, Team CMMD Cycles finished the American Cancer Society's City-to-Shore Bike-a-Thon. Some cyclists on the team logged one hundred miles that day. Together, we have raised nearly $600,000 for cancer research and patient programs.

Inspired by Rachel Platten's hit "Fight Song," a massive group of Team CMMD runners, supporters, kids, and volunteers filmed and released a lip dub video. Not only has this video gotten over forty-six thousand views, but it led to an amazing opportunity for our team. On May 14, 2015, we were invited to attend a live taping of *Good Morning America*. Sixty-six teammates made the two-and-a-half-hour trip to New York City, where we were honored to meet Rachel Platten and the cast of *GMA* and to see clips of our video featured on national television.

One of my teammates was able to deliver one of our team shirts to Rachel, and about a month after the *Good Morning America* appearance, she posted a video of herself thanking fans for making her song number one on iTunes. And what did she choose to wear on that momentous occasion? None other than her Team CMMD T-shirt.

There is no doubt that my journey to Broad Street 2013 was arduous. Along the way, many lives became intertwined. We are professionals, laborers, stay-at-home dads, and single moms, yet our unlikeliest friendships are real and lasting. We have encouraged each other to "just show up" or do "just one more mile." We have lent hands, ears, and shoulders. We have laughed together, cried together, cooked together, and logged thousands upon thousands of miles together. Team CMMD has become a powerhouse of goodness in our community.

Ultimately, my story ends with the person who started it. Tant completed her chemo and had her colostomy successfully reversed. She quickly returned to full-time medical practice, much to the delight of her patients, and began planning a massive wedding celebration for her eldest son. Not only did she appear to be cancer free, but she seemed to be as healthy as ever.

On a blustery January day in 2015, I got a panicked call from my mother. My brother-in-law had had complications following minor surgery and was not doing well. My sister and family wanted me to review his hospital records and make sure everything was being done properly. Over the next hours, faxes and digital reports poured in. I looked over emergency room records, CT scans, and consultation reports. Just when I was ready to render my opinion that all was as it should be, my phone rang again. The caller ID said simply TANT.

The family had called her, too.

"What?" I feigned annoyance, but my heart was full of joy at the sound of her voice. I would never get over my gratitude that Tant had made a full recovery. "Why would they call you, too? I know you're old school and all, but don't they trust me?"

She laughed. "Honey, don't forget *this* old-school doctor made you the good doctor that you are!"

I was crying, and in the moment it took me to catch my breath, she finished.

"I may have made you a good doctor, but you, my dear, are a *great* one."

APPENDIX

For more information about how you can support Team CMMD, please visit www.teamcmmd.org.

View our lip dub video here: bit.ly/cmmddub.

For information about the American Cancer Society and its programs for cancer patients, visit www.cancer.org.

ACKNOWLEDGMENTS

Writing a book is hard.

In fact, even compared to medical school, internship, running a medical practice, and giving birth, finishing this book ranks as the hardest thing I have ever done. Yes, making time to write is not easy—but it was the repeated exposure to this emotionally charged story that I found the most taxing.

This process would not have been possible without the support of my husband, who laughed and cried with me and then scolded me for using the "F" bomb. My three children, Maisy, Sam, and Hadley, endured days and weeks and months of "Mom can't come" and "Maybe later, honey." To them I am eternally grateful.

The book is dedicated to my mom, dad, and aunt, whose stories I tell here. The sacrifices of their generation are what made this possible at all.

The Longest Mile is a story about a team of people. It is those people who make the story what it is. So, to every runner, supporter, and cancer fighter in this story, thank you.

When I needed help choosing the chapter quotes, these teammates—Stephanie Gray, Eric Suchecki, Cari Sobolewski, Claree Nanacasse, Jen Anderson, Karen Moffitt, Kelly Anne Pruden, and Mindy Ellen Ross—came through in minutes with the perfect snippets.

To Judy, TK, Clare-E, and Joan, my coworkers, thank you for being there from the first moment and seeing Team CMMD become what it is today. I am forever grateful to Amy and Tom O'Grady. Without them, the food fight would never have happened nor would it have become the sensation it is now.

Thank you to my sister and my dear friends Kristy and Danielle, who read, reread, and then read again the full manuscript.

The cover photo was created and shot by my friend and Team CMMD favorite, Jamie Stanek. The author photo was taken by Rebekah Ulmer, a woman who inspires me with her resilience every single day.

The publishing process is intimidating. In fact, this book has undergone a complete rewrite. That would not have been possible without my writing coaches, Linda Joy Myers, PhD and Annie Tucker.

Lastly, I have to thank Brooke Warner and everyone at She Writes Press for giving me an opportunity to tell my story. After all, as William Falkner said, "If a story is in you, it has got to come out."

About the Author

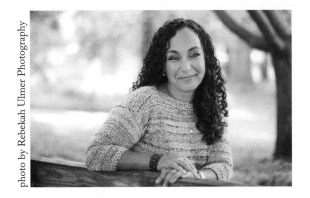

C hristine Meyer, MD, is a board-certified internal medicine physician born to first-generation Egyptian immigrants. She grew up learning about medicine and food from her aunt Venis Fanous, MD. Her medical education took her from rural South New Jersey to the halls of an esteemed medical college in Philadelphia. It was there that she met her husband of twenty years. Together, the Meyers are raising their three children in Downingtown, Pennsylvania.

Dr. Meyer is the founder and managing partner of Christine Meyer, MD and Associates. In addition to practicing full-time, she enjoys writing a blog entitled *Despite My Medical Degree*, which provides a humorous look at the challenges of work-life balance in a two-physician household.

When she is not working, Dr. Meyer enjoys running, cooking, and writing.

In 2012, Dr. Meyer founded Team CMMD Foundation. The foundation's mission is twofold: to support local cancer-stricken families struggling with the financial burdens of their illness and to raise money to fund cancer research.

SELECTED TITLES FROM SHE WRITES PRESS

She Writes Press is an independent publishing
company founded to serve women writers everywhere.
Visit us at www.shewritespress.com.

Renewable: One Woman's Search for Simplicity, Faithfulness, and Hope by Eileen Flanagan. $16.95, 978-1-63152-968-9. At age forty-nine, Eileen Flanagan had an aching feeling that she wasn't living up to her youthful ideals or potential, so she started trying to change the world—and in doing so, she found the courage to change her life.

From Sun to Sun: A Hospice Nurse's Reflection on the Art of Dying by Nina Angela McKissock. $16.95, 978-1-63152-808-8. Weary from the fear people have of talking about the process of dying and death, a highly experienced registered nurse takes the reader into the world of twenty-one of her beloved patients as they prepare to leave this earth.

100 Under $100: One Hundred Tools for Empowering Global Women by Betsy Teutsch. $29.95, 978-1-63152-934-4. An inspiring, comprehensive look at the many tools being employed today to empower women in the developing world and help them raise themselves out of poverty.

The Great Healthy Yard Project: Our Yards, Our Children, Our Responsibility by Diane Lewis, MD. $24.95, 978-1-938314-86-5. A comprehensive look at the ways in which we are polluting our drinking water and how it's putting our children's future at risk—and what we can do to turn things around.

Don't Leave Yet: How My Mother's Alzheimer's Opened My Heart by Constance Hanstedt. $16.95, 978-1-63152-952-8. The chronicle of Hanstedt's journey toward independence, self-assurance, and connectedness as she cares for her mother, who is rapidly losing her own identity to the early stage of Alzheimer's.

Think Better. Live Better. 5 Steps to Create the Life You Deserve by Francine Huss. $16.95, 978-1-938314-66-7. With the help of this guide, readers will learn to cultivate more creative thoughts, realign their mindset, and gain a new perspective on life.